Praise for WHAT I LEARNED IN MEDICAL SCHOOL

"This vibrant collection celebrates the diversity of medical trainees' experiences and brings to the forefront voices too often marginalized in medicine. A testament to the changing face of the profession, this volume reminds both healers and patients that medicine's strengths arise from the rich variety of its practitioners. *What I Learned in Medical School* is the very real humanity of these young physicians."

SAYANTANI DASGUPTA, M.D., M.P.H., author of *Her Own Medicine: A Woman's Journey from Student to Doctor*

"This fascinating collection of experiences underscores the need to implement much higher levels of cultural competency in our medical schools. The book has tremendous educational value and could be used as a catalyst for change."

MAUREEN S. O'LEARY, M.B.A., R.N., Executive Director of the Gay and Lesbian Medical Association

"This book is a must-read for all humanitarians, but especially for medical students of color. The stories in this book speak to the soul and heal while inspiring the reader."

FRANK YONG CHOO AN, M.D., President of the Asian American Physician Association of Southern California, South Bay Region

"*What I Learned in Medical School* should be mandatory reading for all medical school deans."

OMEGA C. LOGAN SILVA, M.D., F.A.C.P., Past President of the American Medical Women's Association

"*What I Learned in Medical School* looks at medical education through the eyes of a diverse collection of students who challenge many of our assumptions about how medicine is taught and practiced. The essays ask us to think about how we measure and treat such differences as race, socioeconomic status, and even weight as part of the identity of the physician—and how a larger, unspoken professional identity has often marginalized many of its members or even excluded a greater richness from its membership."

SUZANNE POIRIER, PH.D., Professor of Literature and Medical Education, University of Illinois College of Medicine, Chicago

"*What I Learned in Medical School* is a ground-breaking coming-of-age-in-medicine book. Each contributor offers a personal and often critical narrative at the intersection of personal identity and the rigidly demanding professional sphere of medical education. This book says more about issues of professional development, and how institutions both thwart and encourage it, than any I've read. These are the issues medical educators should be talking about during whitecoat ceremonies."

DELESE WEAR, PH.D., coeditor of *Educating for Professionalism: Creating a Culture of Humanism in Medical Education*

"This is an insightful and revealing examination of medical education from the point of view of the student. Fascinating and well written, it represents an invaluable addition to the historical and sociological literature on medical education and should be of great interest to general readers as well."

KENNETH M. LUDMERER, M.D., author of *Learning to Heal: The Development of American Medical Education*

WHAT I LEARNED IN MEDICAL SCHOOL

WHAT I LEARNED IN MEDICAL SCHOOL

PERSONAL STORIES OF YOUNG DOCTORS

EDITED BY

KEVIN M. TAKAKUWA + NICK RUBASHKIN + KAREN E. HERZIG

WITH A FOREWORD BY JOYCELYN ELDERS

UNIVERSITY OF CALIFORNIA PRESS
BERKELEY · LOS ANGELES · LONDON

University of California Press
Berkeley and Los Angeles, California

University of California Press, Ltd.
London, England

© 2004 by the Regents of the University of California

Library of Congress Cataloging-in-Publication Data

What I learned in medical school : personal stories of young
doctors / edited by Kevin M. Takakuwa, Nick Rubashkin,
Karen E. Herzig ; with a foreword by Joycelyn Elders.
    p.   ;   cm.
    Includes bibliographical references.
    ISBN 0-520-23936-9 (cloth : alk. paper)
    1. Physicians—Anecdotes.   2. Physician and patient—
Anecdotes.   3. Medical education—Anecdotes.
4. Medicine—Anecdotes.
    [DNLM: 1. Education, Medical—United States—
Personal Narratives.   2. Students, Medical—United
States—Personal Narratives.   3. Cultural Diversity—
United States—Personal Narratives.   4. Prejudice—United
States—Personal Narratives. W 18 W555 2004]
I. Takakuwa, Kevin M.   II. Rubashkin, Nick.   III. Herzig,
Karen E.
    R705.W48 2004
    610'.71'1— dc21

                  2003006769

Manufactured in the United States of America

12 11 10 09 08 07 06 05 04
10 9 8 7 6 5 4 3 2 1

The paper used in this publication meets the minimum
requirements of ANSI/NISO Z39.48–1992 (R 1997)
(Permanence of Paper).

To the thousands of family members, friends, teachers, mentors, colleagues, and patients who helped sustain the individuals in this book. Our thoughts are always with you.

And to the American Medical Student Association for its continued work to advocate nationally on behalf of medical students and patients.

CONTENTS

FOREWORD

When I entered the University of Arkansas in the fall of 1956, I knew that had I tried to go to medical school just ten years earlier, I would not have been admitted. At that time, blacks in the South could attend only black medical schools, of which there were two, Howard University in Washington, D.C., and Meharry Medical College in Nashville, Tennessee. Because of the limited spots, admission to these two schools was highly competitive. Besides, neither had the resources required to run a state-of-the-art academic, research-based institution. Physicians from Howard and Meharry became clinicians in cities and communities; they rarely became professors, policy makers, heads of departments of public health, and certainly not the surgeon general of the United States of America.

But in 1956 a few medical schools were beginning to recruit black students and faculty members. In my entering class, there were three blacks and three women out of one hundred students. Cracks were opening up within the institution of medicine, and indeed in all of American society. As the three of us black students ate together in the segregated cafeterias of the medical school, Martin Luther King Jr. and Thurgood Marshall were organizing marches and rallies around the South.

With the civil rights movement gathering momentum around me, I was focused on my books and stressed over exams. Still, I waged my own small battles with desegregation and built camaraderie with whites around the dissecting table, the microscope, and the hospital bed. I was fortunate to find mentors who took an active interest in my career and development. Racist comments were few and far between, and I never let them pass without rebuttal. I always stood up for myself; I didn't let myself get paralyzed with resentment. What mattered most was completing my degree.

When I graduated, the institution of medicine was far from representative of the American population. The profession was undergoing dramatic demographic and political transformations, and few role models existed for me. I had no way of predicting what kind of career lay ahead. Today, there are more opportunities for blacks and women in medicine. But we have yet to achieve equality for all groups, and discrimination is still a reality for many. Much work is left to be done, and as change continues to occur, the impact on American medicine is unclear.

By sharing their stories, the authors in *What I Learned in Medical School* begin to elucidate the ways in which medicine's new demographic diversity is changing the profession. The writers in this collection challenge us to expand our ideas of who can become physicians and what kinds of careers are possible for these new, diverse practitioners. They narrate the difficulties that arise for people trying to reconcile their differences within a frequently rigid and traditional educational environment. The authors bring a personal dimension to the lives of physicians, who are so often put on pedestals far above "regular" people. Of course, this book is by no means the definitive word on the direction medicine is taking. But it is a starting point for getting to know the new faces in medicine, a starting point for discussion, and, I hope, for action.

In reviewing the testimony and diverse stories of our next generation of American physicians, you get the sense that health care will be delivered in a different manner in the years ahead. Our future health care professionals will understand what it means to be a member of the 5-H club: Hungry, Homeless, Hugless, Healthless, and Hopeless. They will be able to see, hear, feel, smell, and taste the disparities that come with poverty, racism, homophobia, and sexism. They know that we will never have equity and health justice until we understand these issues.

Our new guardians of health know that we must have healthy people in healthy communities, not just the absence of disease. Health is about jobs, education, schools, business, the environment, and diversity. They will make sure that we have a health care system, not just the best "sick" care system in the world. There must be enough room for public health, health education, preventative health care, mental health, primary health care, and reproductive health. We must have a system that is prevention-oriented and available to all people. We need a health care system that fosters an individual's responsibility and human dignity.

The new practitioners must not become equal partners in an oppressive system; rather, they must work to change the system. They can't afford to simply rearrange the furniture in the living room; they need to build a new house. This new house must be big enough to provide high quality care to all our people. It is the responsibility of future physicians to build this system, and they must constantly work to make it better.

Many of you know that health policy and advocacy have been a large part of my career. I feel passionately about advocating for the disadvantaged children of this country. The recent attacks on affirmative action have set us back in maintaining equality of opportunity for the young people of this country, and this includes those who dream, or have yet to dream, of becoming physicians. Nonetheless, I am confident that we will reach the goals of making medicine more representative of American society.

However, complacency is not our friend. As we work from above to keep the legislation and affirmative action structure in place, countless people on the ground are recruiting and inspiring young people to take advantage of the opportunities available to them. I believe that this volume will play an important role in this process of recruiting and inspiring. It is my hope that, with their varied experiences and voices, the authors in this book will become role models for young people of different disadvantaged backgrounds. I have never thought of myself as a role model only for young black women; I hope that my story serves as a source of inspiration for disadvantaged youth of any race or gender. Similarly, I encourage readers of this book, disadvantaged or not, to pay attention to the ways they can be inspired by someone different from themselves.

Joycelyn Elders, M.D.
Little Rock, Arkansas

INTRODUCTION

When doctors are asked what they expected medical school to be like, they often answer with a blank stare. "I didn't really think about it. I knew it would be hard. I just wanted to get in." If asked what medical school was like in retrospect, they frequently say something like, "It was awful. I'm glad those days are behind me."

So what happens to us in medical school? Because prospective medical students are so focused on getting in and on their eventual membership in the prestigious and powerful medical profession, they are primed to be particularly susceptible to the indoctrination that typically occurs. Medical school is, in many ways, like boot camp—patriarchal, militaristic, and designed to strip you of your individuality and turn you into a physician clone, devoid of personality, emotion, or creativity. Your life is hijacked. You're told what to do every minute of the day and overloaded with homework at night.

Always trying to catch up, you devise ways to try to make up for lost time. You shorten your conversations with friends and family until you virtually no longer talk with them. You limit your daily routines until they're unfamiliar. Before you know it, little of your previous life remains.

Your only focus is academic survival. You purge independent thought and don't ask larger questions relating to the educational process: Why does all learning in medical school seem to consist of rote memorization of cookbook-like lists? Why are we so pressed for time that we aren't allowed to ask questions in lectures or pursue in-depth study of interesting medical topics? Why are test scores the only measure of our success? Why does our patient interaction course, where we learn how to communicate effectively with patients, meet only once a week, while hard science courses meet every day?

To ask these questions is to risk losing time that is better spent surviving. Once finished with medical school, new doctors tend to put the experience behind them. For most of us, forgetting the past is a way to avoid examining a difficult or painful process.

So what stories do get told about medical school, and who tells them? Until the later part of the twentieth century, medical schools in the United States actively excluded large segments of the population, including Jews, Catholics, Italians, and other ethnic and religious minorities, especially during the 1920s. For more than a hundred years, it was socially unacceptable for women to enter medicine. Racial minorities were never welcomed. Poor preparatory education and expensive college tuitions limited access for the socioeconomically disadvantaged. Narrowly defined social mores and barriers to the poor meant that medicine as a profession existed for a very specific, homogeneous group of people.[1] Consequently, the perspective of white, wealthy, able-bodied, heterosexual men has generally prevailed. As a direct result of the social, political, and economic changes of the 1960s, however, a dramatic shift occurred in the demographic composition of American medical schools, beginning in the 1970s. But the effects of the influx of a more diverse student population into arguably the most

1. The factors that limited medical education for many are described in K. M. Ludmerer, *Time to Heal: American Medical Education from the Turn of the Century to the Era of Managed Care* (New York: Oxford University Press, 1999), 63–65.

restricted, traditional, and powerful educational institution ever established in America have remained largely unknown.

Since the 1970s, the range of stories about the medical profession has broadened, to include, for example, the publication of memoirs by women physicians and the airing of popular television shows such as *St. Elsewhere* and *ER*, which depict a varied group of medical professionals.[2] Some books have even revealed the once-sacred trials and hazing of medical students.[3] But many of these books were written from the perspective of people with privileged backgrounds, after they were no longer susceptible to retaliation. Many narratives—especially those from the increasingly diverse population of medical students—are still absent. This book is our attempt to showcase their stories.

As we look at the completed book, we believe that it presents a truly wide-ranging collection of stories. It describes how diverse medical students function in what is often still an exclusive, powerful, rigidly confining educational institution that is steeped in decades of tradition and is designed to train only the privileged students of generations past. The students represented in these pages write about why they chose to become doctors, the barriers they faced, the way they view their training, and the struggles they encounter as they progress through medical school. Some students enjoy the new opportunities they experience at relatively progressive medical schools; others struggle in more traditional environments. Each individual also writes with his or her own style and level of maturity. Some authors are directly out of college,

2. Memoirs include P. Klass, *A Not Entirely Benign Procedure: Four Years as a Medical Student* (New York: G. P. Putnam, 1987); E. L. Rothman, *White Coat: Becoming a Doctor at Harvard Medical School* (New York: William Morrow, 1999); and S. DasGupta, *Her Own Medicine: A Woman's Journey from Student to Doctor* (New York: Ballantine, 1999).

3. For memoirs of the "initiation" of medical students, see M. Konner, *Becoming a Doctor: A Journey of Initiation in Medical School* (New York: Viking, 1987); and R. Marion, *Learning to Play God: The Coming of Age of a Young Doctor* (Reading, Mass.: Addison Wesley, 1991).

while others bring their worldly experiences with them. Some are more self-focused, and others are more aware of their relationship to the larger community. Individually, each story can be appreciated on a number of levels: personal, social, and political.

But, taken as a whole, we believe the book accomplishes much more. It documents the struggles of individuals against a powerful institution at a unique period in our history and in the evolution of medical education. It raises questions about how much of our lives we should devote to our work and at what cost to our personal lives. In humanizing medical students and doctors, it leads us to wonder what types of people we want as our doctors and how we can best support them. It encourages us to rethink labels such as "alcoholic," "lesbian," "Muslim," "fat," and "illegal immigrant." It also reminds us that we still do not have equitable treatment for all people, even people in the highest echelons of education. It provokes questions about the effects of affirmative action, immigration policy, and poverty. Perhaps most important, this book may give us hope that, as individuals, we too can overcome great obstacles.

This collection could have included still more perspectives, and we wish we had received an even broader spectrum of stories. For example, the West and East Coasts are overrepresented in comparison with the Midwest and the South, and we received few stories from older students. We were disappointed that we were not able to include some of the important stories that were submitted. Medical students wrote to us about coping with rape, domestic violence, medical student abuse, cancer, and a medical school classmate's suicide. But we required each author to be willing to work with the editors, to have the time to revise his or her story, and to be willing to disclose his or her identity publicly. For some students, these were difficult requirements; consequently, because of busy schedules, an unwillingness to explore deeply personal issues, or a wish to remain anonymous, their stories weren't included. We believed that it was important for each author to be identifiable, in order to be accountable to the truth of the story. With one exception, a woman whose identity as a recovering alcoholic could affect her future career, all the authors allowed us to use their real names. (Note that although the authors are identifiable, all other names used throughout this book are pseudonyms.)

We chose to organize the stories into three thematic sections. Part One, entitled "Life and Family Histories," highlights the unique backgrounds and experiences that people bring with them when they apply to and enter medical school. Eddy V. Nguyen examines what it means to be a Vietnamese boat refugee. His revelations shape his future career goals in medicine. Melanie M. Watkins, a black teenage mother, decides to go to medical school despite huge financial obstacles. During his application process for medical school, Nick Rubashkin struggles with issues surrounding his class background and whether or not to disclose his identity as a gay man. Paul M. Lantos, the grandson of four Jewish Holocaust survivors, contemplates his existence, life path, and career choice. Marcia Verenice Casas crossed the Mexico-California border as a child and reconciles her desire to acculturate into American society with her Latina roots. Heather Goff, a woman with obsessive-compulsive disorder, works to overcome her illness.

Part Two, "Shifting Identities," includes stories about the changes that occur—and the responses they evoke—during the socialization process in the world of medicine. Nusheen Ameenuddin, a Muslim woman who wears a traditional headdress, a hijab, reflects on how her hijab and her short white coat draw mixed public responses. Tresa Muir McNeal is a small-town woman from Texas who moves to a large metropolitan area for medical school and notices how she feels and how she is treated when she returns home. Karen C. Kim discovers that she's considered politically radical in comparison to her classmates and questions why she chose medicine as a career. "Linda Palafox," a recovering alcoholic, hides her identity for fear of repercussions. Rachel Umi Lee delineates the dilemma of trying to maintain her identity as a traditional Korean woman who is expected to "marry well," while also choosing to enroll in medical school and enlist in the navy. Kevin Takakuwa describes his alienation from medical school. Lainie Holman, a lesbian mother living in Ohio, uses humor to describe the absurdities of the medical school curriculum. Anita Ramsetty writes a letter to God, asking for forgiveness for not being a good Christian while in medical school. Akilesh Palanisamy discovers the traditional medical system of India, called Ayurveda, and compares it to Western medicine; he challenges the assumption that Western medicine is superior to other forms.

Part Three, "Confronted," shows how nontraditional students are perceived and treated and how they struggle, internally or externally, to cope, in the face of being seen or treated as outsiders. Robert "Lame Bull" McDonald, a Native American, succinctly describes how a physician he works with views him. David Marcus, a man with Tourette disorder, suffers a lower back injury and is almost dismissed from medical school before he makes a transformation. Tista Ghosh utilizes a standard format for writing medical notes to recall being harassed by a male surgeon. Ugo A. Ezenkwele has an unexpected interaction with a patient and a fellow student. Kay M. Erdwinn contrasts her experiences as a fat woman with those of her classmates. Simone C. Eastman-Uwan chronicles her life in medical school as a woman with sickle-cell anemia. Thao Nguyen (no relation to Eddy Nguyen) presents a graduation speech that was never delivered.

We want to thank the authors for their bravery in exposing their private experiences so publicly, especially in a field like medicine, where nonconformity can feel particularly risky. In presenting these stories, we hope to convey that, on a personal level, we are all unique—and that we need not be ashamed of our differences. On a political level, we hope this book can foreshadow ways in which a dysfunctional system can evolve into something better. Today, medical school admissions are open to many who once were excluded. In comparison to the recent past, medical schools now are made up of more women, underrepresented minorities, and people with disabilities. As our society becomes more diverse, so does the medical profession. By chronicling this change in the demographics of medical students and putting a human face to their stories, we may serve to make these changes more acceptable and may help to shape the medical profession to meet the needs of an increasingly diverse population. Finally, we hope this book brings encouragement both to those who feel isolated as they move through medical training and to brave souls who may be inspired to consider entering the rank and file of a diverse physician population. We dream of a day when we can all be proud to belong to a profession that recognizes and supports the differences among all individuals.

PART ONE: LIFE AND FAMILY HISTORIES

The field of medicine, with its aura of mystique and importance, holds a great attraction. It is well known that many more people aspire to enter medicine than there are spaces in medical school classes. A large number of would-be doctors enter college as "premeds." But the rigorous grading curves of a year of biology, general chemistry, physics, and organic chemistry, the core prerequisites for medical school, cause many to pursue other careers instead. The other major requirement, the Medical College Admissions Test (MCAT), is a standardized test covering biological sciences, physical sciences, reading, and writing. Besides the core prerequisite classes and the MCAT, specific schools may pose additional requirements—for example, a course in calculus. Applying to medical school does not require a particular undergraduate major; applicants may have majored in anything from literature to engineering to business. Once in medical school, however, students with a science background may have an advantage, since much of the course information will already be familiar to them.

Every year, thousands apply for positions in U.S. medical schools.

Currently, there are 125 allopathic medical schools.[1] The percentage of applicants accepted varies from year to year, from 37 percent to 52 percent in the years from 1991 to 2000. During that time, the mean grade point average of successful applicants ranged from 3.45 to 3.60, and the average MCAT score was about one standard deviation above the mean.[2]

In viewing these statistics, it's important to consider at least two factors. First, these numbers reflect the people who actually applied to medical school; they do not include thousands more who completed the required courses or took the MCAT but for some reason decided not to apply. Second, the percentage of successful applicants varies by school and by state. Many state medical schools preferentially or exclusively accept applicants who reside in their state, making their applicant pool smaller and increasing the chances of admission for state residents.

After meeting the basic requirements and taking the MCAT, the prospective applicant files an American Medical College Application Service (AMCAS) application, usually during the summer following the junior year of college. This application is a national standard form for applying to most medical schools. It lists a student's coursework and grades for each semester of college, along with MCAT scores, and includes a one-page essay written by the student stating why he or she wants to go to medical school. The completed AMCAS application is forwarded to all the schools indicated by the applicant. In 2003, the

---

1. Allopathic medical schools, the "standard" form of medical education in the United States, grant the M.D., or Doctor of Medicine, degree. These schools are accredited by the Association of American Medical Colleges. Numerous other forms of medicine are practiced both in the United States and around the world, but for the purposes of this book, we will be referring only to allopathic medicine.

2. For a detailed profile of successful medical school applicants, see *AAMC Data Book: Statistical Information Related to Medical Schools and Teaching Hospitals* (Washington, D.C.: Association of American Medical Colleges Publications, 2001), 8.

application cost was one hundred fifty dollars for the first school plus an additional thirty dollars for each school listed thereafter.

Medical schools then screen these applications to select individuals of interest. Schools send these applicants a "secondary application," which requires each applicant to pay a processing fee and sometimes to provide additional information, often by answering more essay questions. If a school remains interested, the applicant is invited to interview at the campus. The applicant must arrange travel, housing, and food at his or her own expense. The interview usually takes a full day. Applicants undergo a series of meetings with different interviewers (for example, admissions committee members, professors, deans, students), a tour of the campus and facilities, lunch with other applicants and interviewers, and sometimes a financial aid talk with a counselor who discusses the tuition and financial commitment of medical school. Applicants are rated on a variety of factors including academic record, achievements, personality, viewpoints, outside interests, and attention to attire.

Schools then send out acceptances, rejections, and "wait lists" (this last category designating a possible acceptance, depending on how many spaces remain after other applicants have made their decisions). The first acceptances are usually not granted until early winter, and many applicants do not hear a decision until spring or even late summer for classes that start in the fall.

Surviving the progressive narrowing of the applicant pool, and thus gaining entrance into medical school, is an accomplishment. By the time an applicant submits an application, he or she has been invested in the process for at least a couple of years. Hidden behind the statistics of grades and test scores are stories of individuals, each unique, each with a particular set of challenges. The road to matriculation is highly variable. Some applicants are the children of physicians and have had a lifetime of exposure to the profession. Others are from highly educated families and have had the privilege of an excellent preparatory education and a wealth of social connections. Still others are the first in their family to attend college.

The various paths taken to medical school are judged differently. For example, many people assume that it is easier for "underrepresented minorities" (African Americans, Chicanos, mainland Puerto Ricans, Native Americans, Alaska/Hawaiian Natives) to gain entrance because of affirmative action programs or considerations. These assumptions do not account for the additional obstacles many of these applicants have already had to overcome even to be considered for medical school. In contrast, the path of the more privileged is viewed in a different light. It is usually assumed that these applicants are simply hardworking and smart, rather than that they have benefited from social connections, access to private education and tutors, or a learning style suited for medical school.

Affirmative action policies were originally enacted to try to level the playing field for those groups who had suffered historically from decades of discrimination. But the current political tide has moved away from supporting such policies, leaving many to wonder how the profession will recruit and train a physician workforce that will demographically reflect the country's diversity. States that passed anti–affirmative action legislation in recent years (California, Louisiana, and Texas) have seen precipitous drops in the matriculation of underrepresented minorities. This development may also hinder the recruitment of physicians into primary care specialties to work with underserved communities, since emerging evidence suggests that minority physicians are more likely to be drawn to such careers.[3]

In Part One of this book, we present six stories of students with varied backgrounds who took different paths to medical school. The first story is told by an Asian immigrant, who might be labeled a "model minority." Next we hear from a black single mother battling poverty and then from a young gay man who has also been affected by economic

3. E. Moy and B. A. Bartman, "Physician Race and Care of Minority and Medically Indigent Patients," *Journal of the American Medical Association* 273 (1995): 1515–1520, reports these findings.

disadvantage. In another story, the grandson of four Jewish Holocaust survivors contemplates the meaning of his family's suffering and his own existence. In yet another, a woman whose family illegally immigrated from Mexico reaffirms her cultural identity and comes to terms with her ties to both countries. Finally, because demographics are not the only factor that separates traditional from nontraditional students, we include the story of a woman persevering through a mental illness that in the past would have excluded her from medical school if it had been revealed.

These six students, though still young, already have well-developed and distinct identities as they begin their training to become doctors. Their personal and familial struggles not only have given them an enduring sense of identity but also have inspired their decisions to become doctors.

EDDY V. NGUYEN

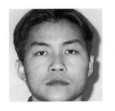

BECOMING AN AMERICAN

Give me your tired, your poor,
Your huddled masses yearning to breathe free,
The wretched refuse of your teeming shore.
Send these, the homeless, tempest-tost to me.
I lift my lamp beside the golden door!

Emma Lazarus, "The New Colossus"

The August 1992 issue of the *Smithsonian* magazine featured an article entitled "The New Saigon" by Pulitzer Prize–winning journalist Stanley Karnow. It documented the new generation of Vietnamese Americans, seventeen years after the fall of Saigon. Beneath the photo of three Vietnamese American students, a caption read, "Refugees Oanh Ha, Minh Tran, and Eddy Nguyen are all honor students at Saddleback High." What may have been another's claim to fame was my humiliation.

Until recently, I would never have mentioned this to anyone. I was ashamed of the image and the caption that branded me, in a conspicuous 11-point Times Roman font, a *refugee*. That word reverberated with my differences from my peers and taught me early on why I could not, and will never be, a bona fide "American." For me, it connoted ostracism and alienation from mainstream culture. In my futile attempt to hide this blemish, I defaced the word "Refugees" in that caption with the thick lines of a black permanent marker. Beneath the layers of ink, I tried to hide my non-American identity.

．　．　．　．　．

When the communist regime took over South Vietnam in 1975, my father was sent to a "reeducation camp" (that is, a prison) because he had worked for the old government. As part of an effort to "deurbanize Saigon," the communists seized my parents' home and forced my family into the "New Economic Zones" to farm for a living. Fearing further persecution, my mother sent me and my sister (four and five years old, respectively) on a boat to Thailand, where we could begin to seek political asylum in the United States, while she stayed behind to wait for my father's release from prison. My journey to America, which took more than a year to complete, took me through the South China Sea, to a refugee camp in Thailand, and finally to the United States, where we had to wait another six months to be reunited with our parents. It was then that I remember meeting my father for the first time.

My family settled in Santa Ana, California, a community with a large number of Vietnamese refugees. I was one of many refugee children who attended grade school alongside white children. In second grade, I had a good friend named Jason. That he was white and I was not mattered little until one afternoon when we were playing soccer on the school field. Somehow, my team consisted primarily of Vietnamese, and the other team was made up primarily of whites. For the first time, Jason and I were on opposing teams.

Much to the chagrin of our opponents, our team won the game. Enraged, they started taunting us, and the resulting exchange led to a barrage of racial insults—they called us "nips" and "chinks" and chanted, "Chinese, Japanese Dirty Knees," and "Go back home where you belong." Along with the words they shouted, they contorted their faces, portraying slanted eyes and flat noses.

Insulted, angry, and hurt, I wanted to protest. We were not Chinese or Japanese; we were Vietnamese. But I knew that it didn't matter to them whether they got the Vietnamese part right or not. The only thing that mattered was that we were not Americans. We were different, and, most important, we didn't belong in "their" country.

Suddenly, I spotted Jason amid the other kids, actively participating in the name-calling and insults. In my disbelief and outrage, I went over and shoved him, accusing, "I thought you were my friend!" He replied, "Go home, nip!" The black eye, scraped knee, and bruised elbow that I incurred from my subsequent fight with Jason were quick to heal. The emotional scar, however, never did.

On that day in second grade, I lost my childhood friend and realized that I was different and would never be accepted as American. As a result, I began denying my refugee identity. Through junior high and high school, at a time when being "in" was so crucial, I spoke little of my experiences as a refugee, fearing that my peers would ostracize me. In class, when a teacher asked about the one childhood experience that had influenced me the most, I never mentioned my refugee journey. When I was asked how I came to the United States, I avoided the truth by saying that I was too young at the time to remember.

.   .   .   .   .

I began college as a pre-med student focused on the sciences. Looking for a break from the routine pre-med classes, I enrolled in a course entitled Art as Social and Political Commentary, which presented artworks from various genres in Western history, ranging from the Holocaust to the Mexican Revolution. The course required a research paper on art as social criticism.

One day, after many hours of flipping through books and journals in my room in search of a topic, I stumbled on a stack of old, dusty magazines. Among them, I came across an old issue of the *Smithsonian* and wondered why I had a lone issue in my possession. Then it came back to me. Curious, I paged to the article, and there it was, the caption that read, "Refugees ... Eddy Nguyen are all honor students at Saddleback High." I could barely decipher the word "Refugees." It was brutally crossed out under aged layers of ink, the markings so heavy that they permeated and tore the page. Seeing this picture and caption for the first time in five years brought back memories of a past intentionally filed away but never forgotten.

At that point, I realized that as much as college had allowed me to grow personally, it had also sheltered me. In college, I was just another Asian among a sea of other Asians. Never once was I singled out as a Vietnamese refugee. Never once was my non-American identity seriously questioned, except in the random acts of discrimination that all Asians likely encounter. Perhaps in choosing to pursue science and medicine, I had deliberately immersed myself in the scientific world of DNA, RNA, and proteins, leaving no time to contemplate the implications of being a refugee. Gazing at that picture brought forth my childhood demons—the name-calling, insults, and shame. I impulsively flung the magazine toward the trash.

But it was too late. The harder I tried to avoid the issue, the more I thought about it. Confused, I didn't know why I felt such an impulse to rid myself of that magazine. And why was I so ashamed of that picture? What exactly about being labeled a refugee was so shameful? Was it the name-calling? Was it the way I tried to speak English in the first grade when I was learning it for the first time? Or was it because my parents never had the time to attend PTA meetings or school functions, as all the other children's parents did? Was it because I didn't get new clothes like the other kids? Was it because my mother never packed a nice lunch box for me the way everyone else's mother did?

Could it be that I was ashamed of being different? But was I really that different? I had mastered the English language, perhaps better than some native speakers. I was about to graduate, with honors, from UCLA and was bound for medical school. While growing up, I had stood by my desk, hand over heart, pledging allegiance to the flag of the United States of America every morning in class. Like my American peers, I had grown up eating hamburgers and fries at McDonald's, drinking Coca-Cola from a can, watching baseball games while eating hot dogs, and listening to the antics of Howard Stern. I, too, laughed at the Three Stooges and cried when the Challenger spaceship fell from the sky or when I saw, even for the hundredth time, footage of the assassination of John F. Kennedy. And I had always rooted for the U.S. Olympic team. But what used to be so clear to me back in high school wasn't so clear any longer. When I left high school and my hometown, I was sure that I also wanted to leave behind the infamy of Eddy the refugee. But now I couldn't figure out why. Why was I different?

These questions prompted me to retrieve the magazine. I stared into my photograph—and for the first time, I read the article that accompanied it. I had found a research topic for my class. I decided to write about the art of the Vietnamese boat people. As I began my research, I discovered pictures of dilapidated boats and squalid refugee camps, along with riveting stories of perseverance, suffering, integrity, and the triumph of the human spirit.

Learning about the Vietnamese boat people through their art and history changed my perspective about being a refugee. Stripped of their homes, possessions, and dignity, many Vietnamese in the mid-1970s believed that they had nothing more to lose and saw only a life of destitution ahead under the watchful eye of the new communist regime. From 1975 to 1985, more than one million of these people fled Vietnam, mostly via overcrowded fishing boats. A large percentage of these refugees drowned or were attacked by pirates and died trying to cross the ocean.

Those who survived sought temporary asylum in nearby countries such as Thailand, Malaysia, and Singapore while applying for refugee status in other countries, including the United States. Despite their dire circumstances, many were later denied the refugee status that would have allowed them to enter the United States or other countries legally, a denial that forced them to return to Vietnam and face persecution. Some, however, chose a different option—the option of suicide—hoping through self-sacrifice to make a bold statement about human rights and the human will to be free.

The images of imprisonment, death, self-immolation, and the struggle for freedom made me understand and appreciate what it meant to be a refugee. One photograph depicted a corporal of the First Airborne Battalion of South Vietnam whose lifeless body is seen dangling alongside the forest trees of Indonesia's Galang Camp. He hanged himself after being denied refugee status, leaving behind a wife and three children. The corporal, who is wearing a red, white, and blue shirt in the photograph, had once fought side by side with American soldiers against the North Vietnamese government. Americans had pledged to aid him in fighting communism, yet when he fled the communist regime to seek asylum in their country, they no longer empathized with his cause. Another photograph contains the image of Vietnamese veteran Pham Van Chau setting himself on fire after he too was denied refugee status. Who was I, then, an ignorant and naïve adolescent, to be ashamed of being labeled a refugee, when others were willing to sacrifice their lives?

A painting entitled *The Black Sun*, by Dai Giang Nguyen (no relation), a surviving refugee, portrays two refugee mothers with forlorn faces and mournful eyes cradling their babies as they stare out from within a refugee camp. In front of them, barbed wire symbolizes the physical and psychological entrapment of the camp. Behind them, a black sun envelops the camp in darkness, representing the bleak prospects for the future of these mothers and, more important, their babies. Nevertheless, in these mothers' eyes a glimmer of hope persists. The trauma of being refugees has not taken away their will to continue fighting for the mere hope of a better future.

These vivid images tell the tales of valiant individuals who chose suffering, the dehumanization of refugee camps, and even death over life amid social and political oppression. To me, they personify dignity, integrity, and the unfettered human spirit.

My research made me realize how ignorant I was to deny the plight of refugees. The calamity of the Vietnamese boat people is not merely the story of those who have suffered, nor is it the story of those who seek pity in their struggle for survival. The Vietnamese boat people are only one personification of the age-old theme of intolerance and persecution of the weak by the strong; remember, for example, the Puritans or the Quakers of colonial American history, who fled persecution in their land of origin. As long as governments exercise absolute power over their citizens and persecute those who are different, there will be refugees.

While reading refugee stories, I vividly recalled my own. I remembered how our frail fishing boat reeked of urine, vomit, excrement, and sweat. I remembered the sound of babies, hungry, crying in their helpless mothers' arms. I remembered the putrid smell of rotten fish that we ate when our food ran out. To reach Thailand, our boat traveled only short distances from island to island in the South China Sea. At each stop, the boat required repairs, and it was always on the brink of breaking down. During our time on each island, we lived in makeshift shacks and ate fish that washed ashore. Once, the boat's engine stalled, and we were stranded out at sea for three days. Adrift and helpless, we were attacked by three different pirate ships. To this day, I can still see a nervous young Vietnamese man with a wooden stick battling a Thai pirate on the deck of the boat. I remember the blue bandana that he wore, drenched in blood oozing from his head.

The gallant stories of my fellow refugees dissolved the shame that I once associated with being a refugee. In college, I began to develop a new self-identity that did not depend on the acceptance of my peers or on how "American" I was. As I developed this identity, I revisited my past and reinterpreted it. At the same time, I had to question why I had chosen medicine. I believe that my parents' experience as refugees instilled in me a spirit of perseverance and the value of education and hard work. Sciences always came easy to me, and medicine seemed like a stable and useful profession. It also symbolized success as an American.

Like many other refugees, my parents left behind established careers that were the result of a lifetime of education and hard work. In the United States, they had to start anew by learning a new language and enrolling in a local community college to learn a technical skill. My father, a successful lawyer in Vietnam, at the age of forty-three faced the daunting task of raising a family while attending classes and working part-time. The only job my mother could get was working as a grocery clerk at a Vietnamese supermarket.

Despite other obligations, my father still found time to tutor my sister and me during nights and weekends to help us catch up in school. My parents eventually took jobs as factory workers at Hughes Aircraft. During my sophomore year in high school, however, they were laid off because of the plant's impending closure. Not wanting to be a financial burden for them, I moved out and supported myself by working full-time at a shoe store. Feeling overwhelmed, I contemplated dropping out of high school numerous times, but my grades convinced me otherwise. My graduation as class valedictorian made me feel that my family's combined efforts had been vindicated.

As a refugee family, we had to work hard, but we also had to learn to accept the help of others in order to survive. I remember in particular a benevolent woman who once provided us with critical aid in Thailand. After my sister and I had been in a Bangkok refugee camp for several months, the adults who had been taking care of us left to settle in Australia. Alone in the camp, we had to fend for ourselves. Fortunately, Madame Yvette, a philanthropic French woman living in Bangkok, came to our aid. She took us home and cared for us for almost a year until we left for the United States. We lived with her two children, and she treated us like her own, providing us with a life of comfort, in contrast to the squalor of the refugee camp. At that time, I didn't understand or fully appreciate her unconditional kindness. We had nothing to offer her. After we left Bangkok, I heard that she continued her efforts to aid the orphans of the refugee camp; she had helped more than twenty refugee children at one point. Her example taught me firsthand the importance of coming to the aid of fellow humans in need.

As I look back on my past, I realize that medicine means more than a symbol of success. To me, it represents the culmination of knowledge and humanitarianism. The change in my life since beginning medical school reflects the self-identity of a refugee, which I now embrace. For the first time in my life, not only am I not self-conscious about being a refugee, but I also feel the desire to bond with and aid the community that I was once ashamed of many years ago.

Before I started the application process for medical school, I thought I wanted to go back east for my medical education. I believed that med school was my chance to venture away from California. I applied mostly to schools on the East Coast, but included a few in California, because my parents would never have forgiven me if I hadn't at least attempted to stay close to home.

Although I received acceptances from schools on the East Coast and in California, I eventually decided to attend Stanford University. One reason was my parents, who constantly nagged me to stay nearby. Another, perhaps more important, reason was my desire to serve in a community where I felt I was needed and where I could really make a difference.

During my visit to Stanford, I spent some time visiting several clinics in the Asian community in the South Bay. Amid the tremendous wealth of Silicon Valley and the "dot-com" boom, I saw an underserved community lacking in basic health care. Many recent immigrants lacked health insurance, either because they did not qualify or because they did not know about the resources available to them. Even for those who had access to health care, there were simply not enough medical personnel to provide this diverse population with culturally competent care. In the Vietnamese community in San Jose, I found out that many elderly patients did not seek medical care for their ailments because they did not want to deal with an "American" doctor. I realized then that my background as a Vietnamese immigrant would be a valuable asset in this community. I felt that I was needed here. Coming to Stanford, all of a sudden, made so much sense to me.

Nowhere else was my experience as a refugee more embraced than during my years in medical school. The flexible curriculum at Stanford Medical School allowed me to spend the time and effort to become involved with the underserved Asian community. The tremendous support from the school's administration allowed me not only to contribute to pre-existing community service programs but also to create my own novel program. While we were planning community health screenings for such problems as high blood pressure and diabetes in the Asian community, my colleagues and I came up with the idea of creating a free clinic for the underserved Asian Pacific Islander immigrant population in the South Bay. We subsequently worked to mobilize the school administration as well as other students to create the first student-run Asian free clinic in the Bay Area.

In medical school, my "American" identity was never questioned, not because it was never an issue but because I chose to embrace the things that were important to me, whether they were mainstream "American" or not. What I stood for and the things I fought for were a reflection of my background and my past. I have long come to terms with my past, realizing that it has enriched my medical school experiences in countless ways.

In the end, to me, being a refugee is no longer about being ashamed of where I came from, how I got here, the accent I might have had, the old clothes I wore, or the pejorative terms used to describe me. It is no longer about fitting into the "mainstream" culture. Being a refugee is about embracing my rich cultural heritage and the experiences that have taught me the value of diversity and giving back to the community at large. For me, medicine is the ultimate application of my experience and my newfound understanding as a refugee.

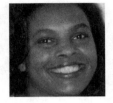

MELANIE'S STORY

I knew for a long time that I wanted to become a doctor. But when I became pregnant at the beginning of my senior year of high school, I thought it would be impossible. After all, most teens who become pregnant in high school drop out and never make it to college, never mind medical school and a three-year residency on top of that.

As a pregnant teen, I felt the judgmental stares of strangers. I lost many of my friends, my boyfriend dumped me, my mother disapproved, and my relatives were disappointed. It was a lonely time.

The loneliest part of my pregnancy was my delivery. I was largely ignored by the obstetrical staff, probably for being just another minority teenager on Medicaid without the baby's father or a family member in the delivery room. The nurses talked about soap operas to each other across my bed as if I were not there. I wanted them to pay attention to me, but as a sixteen-year-old, I didn't feel that I had the power or the right to ask them for anything. I wished I had someone to hold my hand and comfort me, but that person never came.

The delivery seemed like a well-staged play in which I had no role. I noticed the well-timed choreography of the nurses' even-paced steps as they set up the area where the baby would be placed. I saw the doctor's grand entrance. He was masked and gowned in green. I could see little but his eyes, which stared toward my legs and not my face. The lights beamed downward toward center stage, now draped, where the baby would make his arrival.

.   .   .   .   .

With the aid and encouragement of teachers, school staff, and associates of the Howard Hughes Medical Institute, I was able to graduate from high school after the birth of my son and attend the University of Nevada, Reno. Even though I continued to live at home, I had huge concerns about money. How would I pay for school, rent, child care, and food? I applied for food stamps, welfare, public housing, and WIC (the Women, Infants, and Children program)—anything to help pay the bills. It was demeaning to have to apply for assistance, and it was made worse by the time-consuming verification process, during which I was scrutinized as someone who might be trying to "use the system." I remember wanting to apply for scholarships and wanting to work, but I also knew that any such financial assistance would reduce my health insurance benefits and food stamps. I was caught in a vicious cycle.

Though my mother wasn't particularly supportive of me and my son, she did occasionally watch him during my final exams. I got a scholarship from the YWCA for child care and formed a support team with other mothers on evenings and weekends to take turns watching the kids. With the ongoing support of many, including my college professors and staff at the Howard Hughes Medical Institute, I managed to complete my pre-med classes and apply to medical school.

During one of my medical school interviews, I took a hospital tour. I heard one of the doctors say, "I really miss the days of deliveries when a happy husband and wife looked forward to seeing their baby. Now all we have are single women on Medicaid with four and five children." I thought, "Doesn't he know that single women may need even more support? Does he think that none of them look forward to having their baby? Does he think that because they cannot afford a camcorder to record the birth that it is any less important?" I felt an urge to speak out, but I didn't feel it was my place to do so.

His words haunted me for months, reminding me of my own delivery and other encounters I'd had with the medical establishment. For example, when my one-year-old son was evaluated for urological surgery, the doctor spent all of two minutes with us and then scheduled my son for surgery. Later on, I learned that if the doctor had ordered an ultrasound, the surgery might have been avoided. I wonder whether we were given so little attention because I was just another unassertive, black teenage mother on Medicaid.

With age, the responsibilities of motherhood, and my training as a medical student, I began to learn how to assert myself and advocate for my patients in a way no one had done for me. As a volunteer in an obstetrics unit, I encountered a Mexican American woman who did not speak English. I overheard the doctor commenting that this was her sixth baby and that something should be done to keep her from having so many. Meanwhile, the patient was being ignored. I grabbed a towel, moistened it with cool water, and placed it on her head. I offered my hand, and she held it. We were in this together. At her final push, I yelled, *"Bueno! Bueno!"* I did not speak Spanish, but I realized that I did not need to know much of the language to communicate what I wanted to say, to let her know that someone wanted to comfort and support her.

Being a single mother in medical school is not easy. What keeps me going when I am studying at 2 A.M. is not the prestige and recognition that goes with being a doctor, but the promise of a better life for myself and my son and the potential to make a real difference in the lives of my patients. I have shared my story with my classmates and others in the hope that when they encounter a teenage mother, they will consider the difficulty of her situation. Perhaps they will be more likely to respect, support, and encourage her to follow her dreams and plans, as others have sometimes done for me.

I believe that doctors' responsibilities should extend beyond the role of a medical technician; most important, we need to be activists and advocates for our patients. I smile when I think about that day when a young woman will come into my office seeking medical care. She may be scared, alone, and pregnant—but I will tell her that I have been there, and I am here to help.

NICK RUBASHKIN

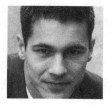

PAVEMENT

I toss and turn on the maroon velour back seat of my uncle's white 1979 Oldsmobile. His sturdy workhorse, this car has registered more than 150,000 miles carrying him to and from his work. Whether I hang my knees over the seat or tuck them against my chest, I can't find a position to suit my six-foot-two-inch frame. In the front seat, my uncle and cousin quietly talk above the traffic report. It's almost 4:00 in the morning, and the report is very short because there is no traffic on the highways between the East Bay and the South Bay at this hour. My uncle leaves precisely at 3:45 every morning to beat the Silicon Valley rush hour, hoping not to lengthen the sixty-minute drive from his home in Oakley to his place of employment, the garage in Milpitas. He works there as a mechanic in his father-in-law's sealing and paving company, Re-Neu Sealers.

A stranger to early mornings since going to college, I have become accustomed to waking in my dorm room, eating prepared cafeteria breakfasts, and just making it to my 10:00 A.M. classes. Grudgingly but gratefully, I'm going to work with my uncle today so that I can borrow the car to drive to Stanford for my last medical school interview. I try to sleep in the back seat because I don't want to be tired as I face the interviewer's questions. It's late in the interviewing season, March 29, and

I'm trying to get a spot on Stanford's wait list. I've been rejected or put on wait lists everywhere else, and Stanford is my best remaining hope.

My options shrank quickly because I could afford only eleven applications. When I filled out the AMCAS application, a general application form for applying to most medical schools, my pen hovered over the box labeled "Financially Disadvantaged." In the end, I did not check it.

Marking that box would have made me eligible for fee waivers. There's a fee for everything in the process of applying to medical school. The MCAT costs almost two hundred dollars; the AMCAS application costs one hundred fifty dollars for the first school, plus thirty dollars for each additional school you apply to; and each secondary application costs at least fifty dollars. Then, if you get an interview, you have to pay all of your own travel expenses—airplanes, hotels, buses, food.

My family was always receiving help. When I was ten, my father was laid off from his job teaching gifted and talented children at five area elementary schools, and we three kids soon received three blue Social Security cards in the mail. Our parents said we needed to get Social Security numbers so that our family could apply for food stamps.

Food stamps look nothing like real dollar bills. The color is different, the size is different—it's as if the government is trying to announce to the world, "This person is on the dole." At the grocery store, my mother would sense other shoppers in line scrutinizing her as she handed food stamps to the cashier, prying eyes trying to make sure that she bought only nutritious, generic items like whole-grain cereals and powdered milk in black-and-white boxes. My mother tells me now that she worried constantly about how she was going to feed me. Always thin, I housed a boundless appetite, shooting up nearly six inches my first summer of puberty. I had a terrible sweet tooth and craved black raspberry ice cream and orange sherbet floating in 7-Up, but ice cream and sherbet were considered luxuries. I grew up wondering why I was always hungrier at other people's houses than at our own.

A few years later, just as my father returned to work and our family began to get on its feet financially, my mother fell ill with a mysterious ailment, which later came to be called chronic fatigue syndrome. She was forced to leave her job at a fabric store and rarely left her bed for the next six months. My father took two jobs: he was a fourth-grade teacher by day, a cashier at a local pharmacy by night. He may have been the only cashier in Maine who held a master's degree in education. My sister and I found jobs that summer, harvesting blueberries to pay for our school clothes. The first Christmas that my mother was sick, unable to do her usual cooking and shopping for the holiday, my father's co-workers surprised my family with full holiday meals and a carload of treats.

A precocious child, I was acutely aware of my family's financial situation. In the year of my father's unemployment, I came to my mother, crying about how we would afford college. She reassured me and told me not to worry. Still, when the time came to apply, we had only enough funds to pay for two college applications.

Yet, aware as I was, my parents protected me and my siblings from the harsh realities of our situation. When I was in college and beginning to explore our family's history, I asked my mother what had been the worst period in our family finances. She told me that when we received the food stamps, we did not even have gas money to go to the grocery store, a twenty-mile round trip.

A product of the things that my parents could not hide and those that they could, I'm confused about the origins and experience of our disadvantage. Were we, in fact, disadvantaged? Disadvantaged compared to whom? And, if we were, do I ever stop being disadvantaged? Where do the effects of family history end and the boundaries of my own life begin?

In retrospect, sometimes it was easy to name. Poverty, if that describes the experience of my family and many of those with whom I grew up, can be loud, insistent, and all encompassing: the force that slams cupboard and refrigerator doors, or the finger that pushes the thermostat down during the winter. (My high school extended our winter break for two weeks during my senior year because the town lacked the funds to heat the building. When we returned to school, we sat in class wearing our winter jackets.) The generalized stress of our financial position erupted at times in arguments over things as small as a magazine subscription; at other times, it surfaced as deep sorrow and shame. (The Christmas he was unemployed, my father cried in front of us because he felt he had not bought us enough presents.) In spite of this visibility, I was never privy to my mother's silent, worried calculations or to the hushed conversations about family finances after we went to bed.

Checking the "Financially Disadvantaged" box on my application would have been so easy in comparison to the alternative I chose, working two jobs the summer before applying to medical school. While other students were padding their applications with internships (often without pay), travel, and research, I was waiting tables and selling clothes. Even with the extra income, however, I ended up using some of my financial aid money to pay for the application fees and travel expenses. Applying to competitive schools on the West Coast was a long shot, given that the travel fund I had accumulated on my own allowed only three bus trips to New York City. I had flown only twice in my life—both times at the expense of other relatives. This time too, I would fly to California only after my father asked his brother Stan, an engineer in Texas, to buy my plane ticket. Even though it was always a last-ditch option, after shifting funds around, seeking out additional job opportunities, and sacrificing basic necessities, asking for help always seemed to mean that we hadn't worked hard enough.

My hesitation over the "Financially Disadvantaged" question belied a host of confusing questions and feelings I had yet to work out about the financial and educational situation of my family. My father, born in Austria, immigrated to the United States when he was two years old. After their arrival in New York, my paternal grandparents moved in with a sponsor family in western Massachusetts, where they found work in factories, my grandfather in a paper mill, my grandmother making toothbrushes. My paternal grandfather died when my father was seventeen, succumbing to a combination of the working conditions in the mill and cigarettes. My father would attend college on the GI Bill.

My mother grew up with eight brothers and sisters in a large French Catholic family. My maternal grandmother, Meme, had been raised in an orphanage and vowed to have a large loving family of her own. She never finished high school because she had to work to support herself and her family. She worked in a shoe factory. Her future husband, my Pepe, was an engineer, the job of an educated person, but they struggled nonetheless to feed and clothe nine children. My mother finished high school and later took some college courses offered through nighttime continuing education programs.

The people in my family have made eyeglasses, cardboard boxes, shoes, and toothbrushes. They have harvested tobacco, potatoes, blueberries, strawberries, and peas. At different times, the family has included store clerks, teachers, nurses, librarians, waitresses, hairdressers, firefighters, foster parents, secretaries, accountants, nursing home attendants, mechanics, cashiers, and soldiers.

In the midst of applying to medical school, I learned that my father's father had once been a medical student in Russia, but that he had been expelled from medical school because of our family's ties to the pre-communist elite. Even in America, he lived in fear of being found by the KGB, and, as a result, I'm led to assume, he humbled himself to live a life that afforded invisibility. Nevertheless, in the factories he was told that he did not belong, because of his smooth hands. My grandmother tells me that the history of this side of the family is like a bottle of fresh milk—from the cow, not the store. Milk separates into cream and the thinner fluid that we drink; our family, she says, has always known both the cream and the milk.

Who am I now that I've tasted the cream? Can I be disadvantaged?

In joyous disbelief on the steps of Harvard for my first medical school interview, tracing my path from a small town in Maine, I wonder at how I inherited a history from a man I never met.

·   ·   ·   ·   ·

The Oldsmobile makes one last turn and comes to a stop, signaling to me that we have arrived. My uncle parks in the yard alongside the inactive sealing trucks, which will be revving up soon. He turns from the driver's seat and gently rouses me.

Groggy, I slide out from the warm car, carefully take my suit from the trunk, and turn to face the garage. It has been eight years since I was last here. The garage looks smaller. Re-Neu Sealers now shares half the space with another sealing company, and the snack machine has been moved to the other corner. The same faded poster with the blonde woman in a neon green bikini hangs on the wall. She smiles seductively and holds a wrench.

Back in 1989, I came to California with my father, who was earning extra income during his summer vacation by sealing parking lots with my uncle. This was the second summer of my mother's illness. One afternoon, my cousin and I swept the garage floor with broad-bristle brooms, trying to earn money to rent video games. For me, it was a summer off; I had spent the previous summer raking blueberries for two dollars a bucket. With the crew of workers, my father spread sealant into the cracks of parking lots throughout the San Francisco Bay Area. The other workers knew that he was a teacher and not a manual laborer. But he told them that when he was on the pavement, he was on their turf. It was his turn to be a student. Classroom, pharmacy, or parking lot—for my father, there seemed to be little difference.

Every day that summer, my father came home with black and crusty hands. He never got that dirty teaching. Somehow, though, he always had the energy to wash up and go with me to the open-air basketball courts in the nearby park. There he taught me how to dribble and shoot and how to fake out the other players. To fake out, you need to have good traction and to move quickly one way and then the other. The lessons I learned on the court had just as much to do with life as they did with basketball: to be successful in either, I would need to be firmly grounded and flexible.

·　·　·　·　·

Startled out of my reverie by the sudden rumble of the paving trucks, I rush to the front bathroom—the clean one, not the one where the workers get changed. I can't get dirty. I check my fingernails; they are still clean. I unzip my suit from the *Time* magazine suit protector that no one in my family has ever used, one of those complimentary gifts that come with a subscription. This is my first store-bought suit. My mother made my first suit by hand, but the seams at the shoulders bunched tightly into ruffles. This jacket, in contrast—forest green, double-breasted, 36 long—looks stunning. It angles my shoulders and cuts my waist. The cream shirt contrasts with the dark fabric of the suit, and the tie adds just enough color. I feel like a pro at putting it on, after wearing it to five other interviews.

In the mirror I straighten my wool lapels. Satisfied with my appearance, I linger, thinking about removing my two small, silver-hoop earrings. I got my ears pierced the summer I came out, but right now, I tell myself, the earrings just don't look professional. It's not that I'm afraid of what the interviewer will think of me. I am queer. It says so on my AMCAS application in 12-point New York Times type: "Coordinator of Lesbian, Gay, Bisexual, Transgender Student Organization, Brandeis University. Two Years."

Dr. Press, a lesbian professor who wrote one of my letters of recommendation, thinks that's why I haven't been accepted anywhere despite graduating magna cum laude and Phi Beta Kappa. I told her about my interviewer at Harvard. As soon as we were done with the interview, he had launched into, "My wife and I just got married and returned from our honeymoon..." Dr. Press nodded knowingly. "Asserting heterosexuality," she said, "is always a sure indicator of how uncomfortable they are."

In or out? I had agonized over that decision when I filled out my applications. I had spent my teenage years in the closet. Now I was too proud and out to even think about going back in. If I tried to hide my sexuality, I would lose half of the activities on my application. I decided to type everything on the AMCAS form: coordinator of my college's lesbian and gay group, my honor's thesis on gay men and masculinity, my coursework on issues in sexuality. And in answer to the question on the application that asked, "What was a particularly difficult time in your life and how did you deal with it?" I wrote about coming out while taking organic chemistry and biology. My personal statement recounted how my experiences shadowing a gay doctor in a free clinic in Boston had clarified my desire to become an activist physician, attuned to the interlocking nature of sexism, racism, homophobia, and economic inequality. After completing my application, I realized that the whole thing was pink.

Now, three hours before my last interview, I hope that being out on my eleven applications doesn't mean being kept out of medical school. Though I'm proud both of being gay and of my family's perseverance in the face of financial disadvantage, the opposite decisions I've made about how much to reveal these identities—to voice one and to hide the other—have surprisingly created a situation where the risk of saying too much and the risk of saying too little become the same.

I tuck my earrings into my pocket and go outside to find my uncle, who has already changed into his blue mechanic's uniform, with a red-and-white name badge that identifies him as "Mike." In his hand, he holds a map that the sealing and paving company uses to navigate the Bay Area. Tracing it on the map, he meticulously takes me along the route from the garage in Milpitas to Stanford. My uncle knows the roads as only a pavement sealer can, and he knows the way to Stanford because his company has done work there.

It's now 6:30, and I'm in a rush to get out of the garage. The workday is starting, and I can't get grease on me. My uncle's hands are still clean when he shakes my hand for good luck. I'm nervous, and I wish he could offer me more than the car keys. Then again, what could he say or do? He's never been inside Stanford. For that matter, what can I offer him in return, me, a queer man wearing his first new suit? I thank my uncle for the map and directions. They get me to Stanford perfectly and easily, where I park the car and step out onto a parking lot that is cracked and needs to be sealed.

PAUL M. LANTOS

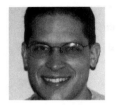

WHISPERS FROM THE THIRD GENERATION

My grandfather would have seen me enter medical school had he lived another four months. A psychiatrist who practiced until his eightieth year, he had been the impetus for my medical aspirations. Like my other grandparents, Apu was a survivor of the Nazi death camps. While each of my four grandparents reacted and coped in unique ways, this grandfather sought solace in medicine. He often credited his knowledge of medicine with saving his life during the war, though we never learned exactly why he felt this way. In fact, he seldom discussed his wartime experiences.

Anyu and Apu immigrated to the United States from Hungary in 1956, when my father was nine years old. The family lived on the grounds of mental hospitals, where Apu worked exceptionally hard. He strongly urged my father to go into medicine, glorifying it as the noblest profession, although my father eventually opted not to become a physician. When I was young, Apu began to encourage me to pursue a medical career. As a child, I enjoyed looking at the pictures in his medical and psychiatric textbooks and copying them by hand. Over the years, he continued to talk with me about his work.

Anyu died when I was thirteen. The night before the funeral, Apu was lying on his bed in the dark. I entered the room and lay on the bed next to him, where Anyu used to sleep. For the next hour, he taught me about Anyu's illness, the reasons for her hospitalization, and the cause of her death. Anyu had been the most overtly sad and withdrawn of my grandparents. She had had asthma, and just as my grandfather channeled his emotion into medicine, his wife channeled hers into illness. She became psychologically dependent on the steroids she took for her asthma, and finally succumbed to the effects of chronic steroid use. I learned much about my grandfather during that conversation. It became clear to me that he truly needed the profession of medicine; its rationality and logic were his refuge from the pain of Anyu's death and, as seems obvious to me now, the pain of his experiences in the Holocaust.

The Holocaust has never been reducible to mere stories in my family. It permeated my grandparents' countenances and in many ways defined their personalities, despite the joy and warmth of their lives after the war. Thus, I understood its importance years before I learned everything that had actually happened. Even when I was very young, it confronted me—when I asked about my great-grandparents, for example, or when I asked my maternal grandfather, Grandpa David, why a number was tattooed on his wrist. For Grandpa David, discussing the war seemed a kind of catharsis. I remember taking walks with him when I was a child. As we walked, he told me frightening and terrible stories about his experiences. I listened, realizing even then that his need to tell exceeded my wish not to hear. He had had nightmares and flashbacks when my mother was growing up, and I often wonder what he thinks of in his most contemplative moments.

Grandma Lola, the youngest of my grandparents, adapted most easily to life in America. Perhaps her adaptability is what has allowed her to philosophize openly about her experiences. She told me about the liquidation of the Lodz ghetto, which happened when she was eighteen. During the deportations, she hid in a pantry with her mother and surviving sisters. They held hands and recited the *sh'ma*, the holiest Jewish affirmation of faith in God: "*Sh'ma Yisrael, Adonai Eloheinu, Adonai Echad.* Hear O Israel, the Lord our God, the Lord is One." By the end of the war, she had lost both her parents and five siblings. She told me that the reason she still kept kosher was to honor the memory of her parents. When I think about her story, I feel a sense of confusion and betrayal directed toward God, and I do not know whether this sense of betrayal is her own belief or mine.

When I was in college, I began to ask my parents and grandparents for more details about the Holocaust. My mother's parents were born in Poland and my father's in Hungary. At the beginning of World War II, my grandparents ranged in age from thirteen to twenty-five years old. Apu spent the war in small forced labor camps. My other three grandparents lived to tell about Auschwitz, but before the end of the war they were transferred to other locations. Grandpa David was marched out of Auschwitz on foot in January of 1945 and survived a death march that lasted until shortly before the war ended in May. He and Grandma Lola were both liberated from Bergen-Belsen and Anyu from Dachau. Six of my great-grandparents were alive at the beginning of the war, but by the end all were dead. One great-grandfather died of starvation in the Lodz ghetto; one survived the camps, only to die in an explosion when he returned home; and all four of my great-grandmothers died in the Auschwitz gas chambers. Many of my grandparents' siblings died as well, most of them in the gas chambers. In addition, one starved, one died of typhus, and one, after whom I am named, was lined up and shot during the Nazi occupation of Hungary.

Survival during those years was as much a matter of luck as strength, and this is obvious in their stories. Anyu's first husband died in the concentration camps. She had had surgery for a tubal pregnancy, and, during the selection at Auschwitz, she realized that everyone with a scar was being segregated with the old, young, and sick. She survived by deftly covering the scar with her hand during the inspection. Grandma Lola went to Auschwitz with her mother, three older sisters, and three younger sisters. During the initial selection, her three older sisters, all in their twenties, were sent to one line, while she, her three younger sisters, and her mother were sent to the other. In the confusion that followed, a Nazi officer, whom she later learned was Josef Mengele, asked my grandmother her age. She was eighteen at the time, but, realizing that being older was better, she lied and told him that she was nineteen. Mengele did not believe her and asked whether she was telling the truth. She still vividly recalls staring into his eyes and insisting that she was nineteen. So he sent her to the other line with her older sisters. When she looked back, she saw her mother and younger sisters for the last time.

My family's history is filled with additional horrifying stories, made infinitely more painful by the knowledge that they happened to my loved ones. Their stories have colored the way I live my life and see the world. At times, they have affected my dealings with patients. For example, when I was doing consultative psychiatry in my third-year clerkship, my team was called to evaluate a patient. He was an old man, speaking incessantly with a strange accent that none of the staff could understand. When I met him, I realized that he sounded like my mother's parents. His accent was Yiddish, and I was able to understand him quite easily. By hiding with a Polish family for most of the war, he had survived the Holocaust and now suffered from post-traumatic stress disorder. Although he was much more impaired than any of my grandparents, it was difficult for me to recognize the man as being ill, because his accent and voice reminded me of Grandpa David. His idiosyncrasies seemed normal and endearing to me, and I felt a strong kinship with him. I therefore found it difficult to have detached clinical discussions about him. After that, I realized that I could never escape my family's past.

As I have grown, my own relationship to the Holocaust has become filled with difficult philosophical questions. The odds that all four of my grandparents would survive were infinitesimal, but I might never have been born had the Holocaust not changed their lives and brought them together. I realize that there is no logic in asking whether my birth somehow justifies the Holocaust. But questions of meaning and purpose have been unavoidable for me. What is the meaning, the obligation, the life path for someone whose birth resulted from the unlikely survival of four people whose families were destroyed? Some people find the answer to this question within Judaism itself. I have been strongly encouraged to marry a Jew and commit myself to a lifetime of model Jewish practice, less because of any merits these actions may have in their own right than because of my family history, which obligates me to pursue such ends.

I do feel a powerful cultural and ethnic connection with Judaism, but my existential bias prevents me from observing devout Jewish religious practices. My understanding of my family's history has, however, imbued me with a great urgency to become a committed humanitarian. I identify the sufferings of individuals and populations with the suffering of my grandparents and their communities. I recognize the continuum of pain and anguish that extends through the past, present, and future of human history. By crusading against the suffering of today, by striving to make up for my family's pain, I feel that I will validate myself. It is to this end that I am pursuing a career in infectious diseases and international health, in which I will devote myself to treating diseases that have individual, social, cultural, and global importance.

Accordingly, during my fourth year of medical school, I traveled to The Gambia, West Africa, for two months, to work in a hospital and participate in research on malnutrition. This symphonic meeting of my professional and philosophical ambitions was not only the pinnacle of medical school for me but also probably the most gratifying experience of my life. The people I met in Africa were extremely warm, friendly, generous, and funny, and most of them lived in appalling poverty. I saw families whose impoverished mother had ten children to feed. I met one mother who has lost five children to AIDS. Children needlessly died of measles, tuberculosis, malaria, dysentery, and AIDS in front of my eyes.

Despite all the tragedy, we were able to save many lives. In my short two months, I saw hundreds of children given a chance to survive to adulthood. Though nothing I do will ever make up for the past evils of human history, I helped give the people of The Gambia something I wish had been given to my grandparents during the Holocaust. I helped give hope, attention, humanity, and life to people. Our patients did not take our care for granted; the father of a severely malnourished child I helped to care for wrote, "Thank you very much for the good help you were for my little child. May God the father of heaven and earth bless you and give you long life and peace so that you can keep helping people." I hope I can continue to help, because even though I cannot save the world, I still have a lifetime to try. But perhaps my greatest hope is that my grandfather, Apu, would be proud of me.

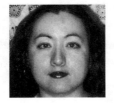

BORDERLANDS

I am originally from Zacatecas, Mexico. My name is Marcia Verenice Casas, and these are my memories.

On any given day, Latino Indians swim across rivers and hide in crowded, rotting trucks as they cross the Mexico-California border. It is a simple border, drawn in barbed wire and metal fence, separating two peoples, two cultures. Human beings risk their lives for the chance to work at Jack-in-the-Box; they risk death for the chance to wash some white guy's BMW for a dollar tip. They risk it all for that elusive American Dream.

I am a little girl again, and it is bitter cold. We are hiding in the shadows of Mexico's hills near the border, trying to stay away from the probing lights of the immigration trucks ahead. I hear the helicopters swarming above and feel their searchlights burning holes in my clothes. I crouch even lower so the border patrol won't see me. They are so close I can hear their strange English words. My clothes stick to my skin, and I bite my lip to keep from crying.

I am being hunted. What will happen if we are caught? Will they kill us? Or send us back? But we can't go back. I squeeze my eyes shut so tightly I think I will go blind, and I pray to God that we are not caught. I think of my grandmother, *mi abuela* Concha, who stayed behind in

Zacatecas because of a sick heart, and the thought of her calms me somewhat. Suddenly, the voices ahead subside and the lights move away, and we begin to creep toward the shining lights of San Diego. Then I am running, running like the wind so as not to be left behind. This is all I can remember of that time.

My family and I settle in a small town near Sacramento, California. There is more work here than in Zacatecas, and my parents take many jobs to feed us, their three children. It is hard work: farm labor in 100-degree heat, canning tomatoes hour after hour, washing dishes and floors, and hammering away at new houses for people who can afford a price tag that makes my eyes open wide in disbelief.

Here in this rich new country, I am embarrassed by what I do not have. Why must we live in a shack? Why do I have only two pairs of pants? I am envious of my rich classmates who wear fancy new clothes, whose parents bring them to school driving shiny new cars. When my father finally buys an old rusted truck, I am so ashamed that I ask him to drop me off two blocks from school so no one will see it. When a classmate's mother offers me a ride home one day, I tell her it is *that* house in the suburbs, the one on the right with the white picket fence. I wait for them to round the corner and then proceed to walk the five miles to my real house in the barrio.

At school, I find that I pick up English quickly. I love to learn and am in awe of books. I cannot wait for the library to open in the morning so that I can sneak in another half hour of reading before school. I find myself reading most nights as well. My father tells me to read as much as I can. And I do. I read books, magazines, even the backs of cereal boxes, milk cartons, and the soda cans my mother picks up from parks to recycle for extra income. I hide in the corner of the school library and use my Spanish tongue to sound out the odd and clumsy English phrases.

But no matter how much I practice and study, my white classmates whisper, "Where is she from?" Others yell, "Go back to Mexico, wetback!" The word, I come to learn, refers to our soaked clothes when we swim for our lives across the river at the border. When I mention to my father that I have been called a wetback, he turns to me and says, "Be proud of your culture. Remember where you come from. Stand by that which you believe." But I wonder what he is talking about. What culture? I turn back to my books and begin to think my father is a crazy old man who does not know what he is talking about.

But reading and learning English do not mean that I fit in. I refuse to speak Spanish anymore, deciding to do whatever it takes to feel accepted. I choose to become like them, like the white kids who belong to the majority, who laugh at the new immigrant kids who speak only Spanish. When a teacher asks me how I pronounce my name, I tell her, "Marsha." My siblings do similar things. We all speak only Anglo, even to our parents. We all dress like the white kids. We all deny our Latino heritage any way we can.

New Latinos, recent immigrants, enter our classes almost daily. They try to meet my gaze as I walk down the hall, and I sense the *"Hola"* on their lips. I look away. How dare they speak to me? I am embarrassed that they think I am like them. Latinos who aren't new look at me with disappointment. I hear their whispers: "Sellout!" "Whitewashed!" I am not like them. I will not be. So I pick up my books and keep reading.

And slowly I begin to be accepted by the white kids at school, who look at me as some kind of exception. They start to say, "You're not like them." They mean, of course, that I am not like the other Latinos— dirty, lazy, dumb people good only for manual labor. I am ecstatic, not angry, at the slur, because now I realize that some of my classmates no longer think I am a wetback. But I know that inside I am uncomfortable. I feel I am in some borderland, somewhere between this white, American world and the other Mexican one. I do not understand why I feel this way. But I do not wish to.

My need to assimilate affects my life outside school too. I stand in line one day at the grocery store. Next to me is a Latino man who looks like he has just gotten off work in the tomato fields. The white cashier tries to explain to him which coin is a quarter, which a dime. The man turns to me with a pleading look, asking in broken English if I speak Spanish and can help him. I turn away and say in my best English, "No, I don't speak Spanish." I feel my face turn crimson. Do the other customers see him talking to me? I pray they do not think he is my father. But I also feel something else. Conflict. Why am I so ashamed of what I have just done?

The incident reminds me of another time, when my father asked me to translate for him at the free community clinic. I was ashamed to be seen there, because everyone knows that if you go there you are poor. But he is my father, and so I went to help him. He had just gotten off work. He was building houses, and his pants were torn and soiled with white paint. His hands were callused and dry from laboring in the searing heat. As I sat next to him in the waiting room, I felt my face getting red from embarrassment at how he was dressed. I saw the white receptionists glowering at us as if we did not belong there.

The doctor who eventually saw us would not touch my father's hands. He asked my father to wash his hands. My father explained that the water had seeped into the cuts on his hands, and it ached too much to wash them. The doctor acted offended. He made a point of greeting the next patient, a well-dressed Latino gentleman in shirt and tie, with a firm handshake. My father gave me a knowing look and held his head high.

Now, at the grocery store, I remember that time. How dare that doctor humiliate my father? This is the first time in my life when I realize that something is not right.

But I am still embarrassed by my father. When I receive an academic award, he arrives at the ceremony a little late, because he has rushed there from work. He's still in his work clothes. The other recipients all ask their families up to the stage to thank them for their support in front of everyone. I cannot bring myself to do it. I thank my parents from afar, where they sit in the darkened auditorium. Later on, I cry in anger at myself. My father has again been insulted, and I cannot believe that I was the one who did it.

Other events slowly stir my Latino consciousness. My father declines to go on welfare and take food stamps. He refuses to be another Latino taking "undeserved" money from the government. So, on the days when there is not enough food, my mother goes without. I feel helpless, convinced it should not have to be this way. My father always tells us that education is what matters, but so does family. My brother and I begin to work as well as go to school. Family is as important as getting good grades and assimilating.

Late one night, I sit at the kitchen table after work, doing my homework. I read the assigned novel *Like Water for Chocolate*. To my astonishment, I love this mystical story about a Mexican family's adventures in life and the foods they cook along the way. A few weeks later, I ask my mother if she will teach me how to cook some of the dishes in the book. She is surprised by my request; I have never before shown any interest in *su tierra*, her land. I think I am surprised, too.

Another time, I drive to the tomato fields to pick up my mother from work. At first, I crouch down in my father's truck because I do not want to be seen there. But my mother is not waiting for me, so I have to go into the fields to look for her. To my left, I see an old man hunched over the plants, barely able to move. To my right, a pregnant woman holds her belly with one hand and picks tomatoes with the other. She tells me that she has never seen a doctor because she has no money. She is illegal. I look, really look, now at the other workers. They all look the same, with bandanas over their faces to protect them from the dirt and pesticides. I am suddenly filled with guilt. They look like my father, like my mother, like me. My shame has betrayed someone, something, although I cannot yet explain who or what. I am frightened. I hurry my mother to the truck and drive away as fast as I can.

The academic counselor at school recommends that I take home economics courses. The school tells my brother that he needs to take special education classes. He speaks with too much of an accent, and all he does is draw—on paper, on the boards, on the desks—so he must be slow. My mother refuses. Even so, I think my brother is haunted for years by this incident. Meanwhile, I watch nature and science programs on TV and am intrigued. I want to learn about math and science and become a doctor someday. I decide to tell the counselor this, sure that he will encourage me. I say I need to go to college and must take the right courses to prepare. I explain that my parents never had the chance to get an education and that I want to honor myself and them by pushing forward.

But the counselor looks at me with pity in his eyes and a half-smile on his lips. He says that I should just concentrate on graduating from high school. After all, that would be a step up from my parents. Perhaps college could be for my children. I am crushed. After all my work, all my efforts to become American, I suddenly realize that for this man I am still just an immigrant. I mutter, "Okay, thank you," but I register for the courses I want anyway.

In a school full of Latinos, I am the only one in these honors courses. I am determined to succeed, and I study for hours. It is difficult with no one at home to help me; no one in my family knows anything about algebra, let alone the other classes I need to get into college. I do have one teacher, though, a white chemistry teacher, who pushes me. He tells me I can do anything I want, and I am fueled by his encouragement.

At the same time I am increasing my appreciation for academic achievements, I am losing the need to use them as a means to be accepted. Slowly, I feel the importance of assimilating give way. I notice that in my world history class I hear only about white people. All the heroes of diplomacy and democracy, the teachers imply, are white. I am taught only about Europe and the United States: European philosophers, white intellectuals and humanitarians, and American freedom fighters. It is as if I and all my people have contributed nothing and indeed are nothing, because we are not white.

I meet a new friend, Samuel, a Native American. His mother invites me and my siblings to visit them in Point Reyes, with its huge redwood trees shooting up into the sky. Samuel's mother tells us that we must respect the land, that it belongs to no one. She tells us that Columbus "discovering" America is a lie. There were people, our people, living here, with their own civilizations, long before the European armies arrived. She tells us to be fearless and never to forget that these native people are our people. She says, "Have dignity for yourself. Remember your roots." I leave Point Reyes with memories of whales swimming in the Pacific waters, a tent filled with steam and sweating bodies, and the huge trees whose leaves stretch closer to my beloved moon than I ever will. And I leave Point Reyes still confused about myself and my "roots," but now I am thinking hard. What did she mean?

Once again, I stand in line at the store, this time the local 7-Eleven. The Latino man next to me is having trouble figuring out the change, just like before. The Latina cashier looks at him with annoyance, and it makes the blood rush to my face. I help the man and then turn to the cashier. "Don't think you're something you're not. Don't think you're better than he is because your English is better." She looks at me like I am crazy. I rush out, almost expecting her to follow me and kick my ass. And yet I am smiling.

I finally realize that I have roots. I have been aching for them all these years since leaving Mexico. I return there to visit before I begin college. It has been seven years. What will my relatives think of me now? Will I be able to speak Spanish without sounding terrible? Sure enough, my relatives call me *"Pocha"* (whitewashed) and *"Gringa."* Not American enough in America, and now not Mexican enough in Mexico.

But for the first time in my life, I do not care. I am becoming sure of my identity, and I laugh right along with them. And I notice that my Spanish words flow with an authentic rhythm I have never heard in myself before. I hear my name pronounced as it is supposed to be, with the accent on the first syllable, and I love how it sounds. I soak up the culture, the traditions, the foods—my roots. On September 15, Mexico's Independence Day, the entire town turns out, and the plaza is filled with loud music and banners of red, white, and green. I have never felt such peace. I am home.

During my visit, I have long conversations with my aunt, asking her about *mi abuela* Concha because my father refuses to speak of her. He adored her so much that he cannot imagine her dead. I learn that Concha was a beautiful Indian woman, with dark, creamy skin that felt like velvet. She suffered most of her life with "heart trouble." But she blessed our move to California, telling my father that she would be fine staying back in Mexico. She always insisted to her children that she was well, even as her doctor told them to pray for her, and the priest held a cross to her forehead every time she fainted. I listen to my aunt tell the story, and I can barely stand to hear another word. I cry, wishing that I had known her better and that she had not suffered all her life. I have wanted to be a doctor since I was seven, but now I begin to think of being a healer to people like Concha.

When I return from Mexico, I begin college, now firmly connected to my roots. I speak only Spanish with my family and tell people how to correctly pronounce my name. I volunteer as a tutor for migrant children, encouraging them to follow their dreams, and I become a role model of a proud Latina pre-med college student. Once a year, I return to Mexico. Now I wear a necklace I bought in Zacatecas, engraved with the calendar of the Aztec people, my people.

My fifteen-year-old sister, who has a much stronger Latina identity than I had at her age, is starting her high school's first M.E.Ch.A. chapter—an organization dedicated to increasing cultural awareness, pride, and equality for Chicanos and Latinos in education. She has always been involved in politics, especially concerning the rights of immigrants. Whereas before I had always brushed aside her attempts to engage me in political conversations, I now listen with interest to her ideas about eliminating racism and increasing equality for everyone. It is 1994, and I begin to hear about California's Proposition 187, an anti-immigrant proposition that would deny health care to immigrants and education to their children. I watch the propaganda ads on television depicting Latinos in long lines at the welfare offices and crowded into waiting rooms at free community clinics. The people of California are taken in by these ads and vote for Proposition 187. The proposition is immediately challenged in the court system as unconstitutional.

I work at the local community clinic—the same one I visited with my father years ago—and neither the doctors nor the patients are sure of what to do. Under the new law, doctors would be required to report illegal aliens and deny them health care. The patients, desperate to see a doctor, are terrified of deportations and wait tentatively for hours outside the clinic. The doctors and staff meet. During the discussions, I ask aloud whether there's even a mention of "illegal aliens" in the Hippocratic Oath. Eventually, we decide to treat everyone as we usually do.

We have a Latina neighbor whose parents crossed the border years before she was born. One day she smiles and waves at me across the lawn, telling me she has voted for Proposition 187: "There's no way my tax dollars will go for medicine for any wetbacks!" In almost the same breath, she continues, "I'm so glad you're going to become a doctor." It is obvious she has forgotten what her parents sacrificed to make a better life for her. I decide to speak up. "I crossed the border when I was little." It feels good to assert who I am.

It is the end of my last year of college. After my graduation ceremony, we have a beautiful Chicano/Latino celebration. The graduates each have a few minutes to speak. This time, I invite my parents up to the stage, and, in front of hundreds of people, I pay homage to their struggles and the encouragement they have always given me. It is only the second time I have ever seen my father cry.

I am in my second year at Stanford University Medical School. I decide, after much deliberation, to apply for a $75,000 scholarship for "New Americans." I am hesitant because I know what I have to say to win it; someone who won it in the past has warned me. I need to portray a fully Americanized person. After years of learning to embrace my cultural identity, now I will have to deny it. I am a finalist, and they fly me to Los Angeles for the final interview. I wonder whether I can act the part of an "assimilated" girl for one hour. But the scholarship means that

I could leave medical school with no debt, and it might afford me the chance to work at a community clinic serving uninsured immigrants. I have to do this. So I practice how it would feel to say, "My name is Marsha; I have given up my roots for a better culture; I choose not to speak Spanish anymore; I have no plans to return to Mexico." It feels bitter to my tongue.

I stay for free in a beautiful hotel in Los Angeles. As I walk around, I see Latinas in their maid outfits cleaning rooms and scrubbing the floors that I step on. Latino bellhops carry rich people's bags. I feel that I am bearing the weight of every Latino I have ever known. "I can do this," I keep telling myself.

The interview is awful. I hate myself as I lie about everything I believe in. Finally, one of the panelists asks, "Marsha, what do you believe in as a New American?" In a split second, the memory of my father's words strikes me: "Stand by that which you believe." And I suddenly know that I cannot lie any longer. So I face the panelists and calmly say, "I believe in bilingual education. I believe in affirmative action for inner-city youth. I believe in holding on tightly to a sense of cultural identity, no matter where you live. And, by the way, my name is Marcia, not Marsha." They look at me as if I am crazy, and I can feel the money slipping through my fingers. I know I will not get the scholarship. But I know also that I can look at myself in the mirror and speak the truth, that I stood for that which I believed.

. . . . .

I am now in my third year of medical school. My sister, a former gang member turned political activist, is in law school. My brother is completing a master's degree in art; he draws wondrous murals of the Mexican Revolution and scenes of Latino children. My mother is a housekeeper. My father is a common laborer.

HEATHER GOFF

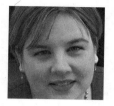

POISON IN MY COFFEE

uring my first year of medical school, I took a class called Behavioral Science and Psychiatry, a required course that covered child development, drug addiction, sexuality, and psychoses. One day in class, the professor mentioned that 2 percent of the U.S. population suffers from obsessive-compulsive disorder (OCD). There was an immediate flurry from members of the class, as they quickly calculated the implications of such a statistic.

The student next to me leaned over and whispered, "That must be wrong. Two percent? That means four people in our class have it. That's impossible!"

I smiled ironically. Little did he know that I am one of the reputed four.

It all started shortly after college, when I began believing that my coffee was poisoned. I would contemplate each cup until it became too cold to drink. Gradually I began to believe that all my food was poisoned. These thoughts triggered several panic attacks each day. I also started finding it necessary to watch the movie *Clueless* in its entirety before I left for work each morning. Then I had to watch it again when I got home—and again before I went to bed. Then one day I suddenly started to cut myself with a single-edged razor blade. Cutting seemed to make all the obsessive thoughts go away, so it quickly became a necessary safety valve.

My symptoms became so debilitating that I sought out a psychiatrist for the first time in my life. I didn't particularly like him, but each week I would dutifully arrive at my appointment. He would usher me into his office, and I would sit in a chair he had placed directly opposite him, which allowed me no escape from the cold, lifeless gaze he had perfected. He would ask how my week had been, and, like clockwork, I would reply, "Fine." Then silence. Reticent by nature, I had difficulty figuring out what I was supposed to talk about.

Sometimes I would tell him that I hadn't eaten a complete meal in two days because I was terrified that my food was filled with some deadly substance. He would then inform me that I really should try to eat regularly, but he offered no insights or suggestions about how I might do this. When I finally mustered the courage to tell him about cutting myself, he told me to throw out the razor blades. We did not discuss why I might be hurting myself.

I saw this psychiatrist once a week for a year. Throughout this time, my diagnosis remained unchanged: "Stressed out." I once asked him what most of his other patients complained of. "Misery," he replied. "General life unhappiness." Unfortunately, he seemed to have only one diagnosis, and I didn't fit it.

He did at least give me antidepressants. The medication seemed to help a little, but not enough, and therapy with him didn't help at all. Unknown to me at the time, and evidently to him as well, I suffered from OCD along with my clinical depression. But he was my first psychiatrist, and it somehow didn't occur to me then that a patient who doesn't like a doctor can look for a new one.

Finally, after months of trying to convince him that I was ready to leave therapy (I really just wanted to leave therapy with him), I started looking for a new psychiatrist. I found a wonderful doctor in less than a month. Fortunately, she was familiar with the symptoms of both depression and OCD. I finally had a real diagnosis that made sense to me. At last someone could explain what was happening inside my head. I learned that, like many other "cutters," I wasn't adept at expressing strong emotions like anger and sadness. Instead of addressing my feelings directly, I was using my own skin as an outlet for them; and my obsessive, irrational fears at times exacerbated the cutting.

With the help of my new doctor, I slowly learned how to deal with those emotions in a more productive manner. I started talking to the people who evoked strong emotions in me rather than "talking to" my own arms. We also experimented with various types of medication and different dosages until my depression started to lift and my obsessions slowly waned. Eventually, I didn't feel as compelled to cut myself anymore.

During this admittedly rocky time of recovery, I heard that I had been accepted into medical school.

I'd been thinking about medical school for years, on and off. During college, I took the MCAT and the required courses, but I didn't apply right away because I wanted to be absolutely certain that I was applying for the right reasons. My father is a doctor, and although he never once pressured or pushed me, I wondered whether, at some level, he was truly the reason I wanted to be a physician. I decided to take a year or two to work in clinical research, to gain some perspective and experience.

But then one day, I realized that it didn't matter why I wanted to be a doctor, whether it was partly because of my dad or partly because I loved science. I simply knew that I didn't want to go through life without learning more about what makes humans "work." I didn't want to go through life without reading medical journals. And clichéd as it may be, I really did want to help people. That realization, along with my work in clinical research, pretty much sealed my fate. I knew I'd found my calling, despite the obstacles that were to come. And so I had finally applied to medical school.

How I managed to get accepted when I was barely able to get up in the morning is still a mystery to me. Luckily, I had filled out the first set of applications during an upswing, when I was feeling pretty good about life. I had even outlined answers to questions often posed in secondary applications and interviews. When the depression hit again, I simply copied down my previous drafts on the secondary applications, and when interview invitations arrived, I was ready.

In the midst of a giant downswing in my mood, I went to my interviews dressed in a sweater set. I didn't have the energy to buy a suit. Oddly, this may have actually worked in my favor. At least I stood out from the rest of the day's applicants—I was the only one not wearing a dark blue suit.

I trudged wearily behind the other applicants during the tours, but when it came time for the actual interviews, I somehow pulled myself together and drew from my acting classes and experience: I smiled, looking eager and animated, just like a medical school hopeful should. At the end of the interview hour, I was exhausted from the effort and wanted only to go home and crawl into bed until the next school's interview.

I don't know whether it was my smile, or perhaps the sweater set, but by May I had received two letters of acceptance and three wait list positions. I had made it into medical school. And depression, OCD, and self-mutilation notwithstanding, I'm still here.

Since I first began treatment for OCD and depression, I've been engaged daily in a Hamlet-inspired debate inside my head: to take or not to take medication. I have learned, however, that medical school is neither the time nor the place to experiment with self-imposed treatment termination.

At the start of the winter semester, I had missed a few weeks of therapy amid the flurry of exams and holidays. At the same time, I finished the last of my Prozac. Instead of getting a refill, I decided to stop taking it. I ended up in bed, where I stayed for a month. I simply slept. I failed all my exams that month, but that didn't worry me. Nothing really worried me. I was too depressed, lying in bed and cutting up my arms, to get nervous about things like my academic standing.

Why would anyone stop taking their medication, given the severity of OCD symptoms? I've asked the same question of other patients. Treatment compliance is always an issue in any type of patient care. In psychiatric care, the problem is compounded by cultural beliefs and the stigma surrounding mental illness. Although intellectually I understand that antidepressants treat brain chemistry in the same way that insulin treats blood glucose chemistry, on an emotional level I have great difficulty coming to terms with taking psychiatric medications. It's one thing to take antibiotics because you get an infection. The infection isn't your fault; it can happen to anyone. But taking medication because you feel "sad" all the time makes you suspect that something is wrong with *you*, not just your chemicals.

When I started taking Prozac three years ago, I felt like a weak person for taking medication to improve my mood rather than just dealing with my unhappiness the way most people do. What I missed, however, was that my unhappiness was not the same as most people's. I didn't understand that my sadness, anxiety, and obsessions all stemmed from a serotonin deficiency in my brain, not from a problem in my social life or my character. In the same way a person with diabetes takes insulin to correct a glucose imbalance, I must take Prozac to correct the low levels of serotonin in my brain. But unlike diabetes or an infection, conditions whose symptoms are physical, depression and OCD have symptoms that are mental and emotional. How can an imbalance in neurotransmitter levels make me believe that my food is poisoned? How can it make me feel so sad that I cry for hours at a time? The concept is difficult to grasp, and I struggle with it every day. The evidence for the benefits of antidepressant treatment is obvious: I feel normal when I take medication and abnormal when I don't. I'm slowly catching on.

During that winter semester of my first year, under threats from my parents and friends, I finally dragged myself back to my psychiatrist. I restarted the Prozac, and when enough time had passed for me to feel its effects (about another month), the seriousness of my situation hit me like a Mack truck. Only three weeks left in the semester, and I was failing every class.

There was no way to catch up. I met with my professors. I met with the dean of students. I considered taking a medical leave of absence. I considered repeating my first year. In the end, my physiology professor suggested that I forget about physiology and concentrate on biochemistry, neuroscience, and behavioral science. I would have to retake physiology over the summer. Luckily, biochemistry had been my undergraduate major, so I was able to pass that class. And I somehow made it through the other two courses.

It was in the middle of the behavioral science class that I listened to the guy next to me declare the absolute impossibility that four of his fellow students were suffering from OCD. There I was, "learning" about OCD and trying to remain objective about something that has been my personal hell. There I was, "learning" about depression and trying my hardest to convince myself to take my own antidepressants.

Scientists are supposed to look at information with a clear eye and an open mind. As physicians-in-training, we are supposed to listen to patients' problems in that same objective manner. But how do I do that? How can I sit and listen to a depressed patient without remembering some of my own pain? How can I watch a patient with OCD go through a compulsion and not be drawn to my own compulsive behavior? We are taught not to discuss ourselves, not to give out personal information to our patients. But as a patient, what wouldn't I give to hear someone say, "I've been there too. I understand. I got better, and so can you"?

The reality is that I probably won't advertise my mental illness, but I can give out information about myself on a need-to-know basis. I think that after medical school I want to specialize in psychiatry. Sometimes I'm not sure that's such a great idea, given my own mental health history. But part of me feels like psychiatry and I fit together, like it's just what I'm supposed to do. Maybe I got sick for a reason. On my good days, I'm convinced that my future patients will benefit from my ability to empathize with their experiences.

I still have difficult days. Sometimes I don't want to get out of bed, and I'm not sure whether it is depression or the pathology exam looming at 9 A.M. Sometimes I make my friends taste my food, and I'm not sure whether I'm being obsessive or generous. My friends are for the most part supportive, although they get a little tired of my more irrational fears. But, overall, I am getting better. Some days I forget that I have OCD; and with medication, I have been symptom-free for quite a while now. My doctor cautions that my symptoms will probably come back, but when that day comes, I'd like to think that I will know what is happening inside my head and how to fix it. Today I understand that, while my experiences with OCD and depression undoubtedly have shaped me and the physician that I will become, they are only a fraction of all my life experiences. I am more than just a psychiatric patient. And I am more than just a medical student. I am me.

PART TWO: SHIFTING IDENTITIES

Once in medical school, students face a shocking new reality. Whether by design or evolution, medical school delivers a constant barrage of information. Typically, the first two years, called the "pre-clinical" years, are devoted to lectures and laboratories covering the basic sciences. Subjects such as anatomy, biochemistry, and pathology are among the most rigorous. Others include physiology, microbiology, pharmacology, endocrinology, hematology, cardiology, pulmonology, gynecology, obstetrics, and a patient interview/physical exam course.

Keeping up with the extremely rapid pace pushes most students beyond any limits they might have previously experienced. Lectures superficially cover incredible quantities of information. For example, a week of lectures may cover an entire semester of college-level physiology. The rules of learning that became familiar in college no longer apply. A lecturer might mention muscle mechanics but doesn't have time to cover the details of how it works. A medical student might not know that the lecturer now expects the student to go home and independently learn the details.

In college, professors tend to allocate lecture time proportionately to what students are expected to learn, but this doesn't happen in medical school. Lecture classes rarely allow time for questions or discussions. Socratic methodology is completely absent—there's no time. Everything is laid out, with no room to deviate. With four to six classes in one day, it's clear that most students can become overwhelmed with information. To add to the pressure, professors frequently assign other tasks: weekly quizzes, question sets, papers to write, and additional readings. But simply reading the assigned textbook pages at an average pace would keep a student busy for more than twenty-four hours a day, seven days a week, for the entire semester. Somehow, the student must learn what the professor deems important and unimportant. The way most students cope with the myriad requirements of the pre-clinical years is by studying very hard for long hours, all the time, at any cost.

Usually at the end of the pre-clinical years, students take the first of three "Step" tests from the National Board of Medical Examiners. Failure to pass Step I generally means that a student cannot progress to the "clinical years" (the third and fourth years of medical school). The failure rate is set at approximately 5 to 8 percent of those taking the exam. Because of this built-in failure rate, passing Step I is a source of extreme anxiety, and some schools have even altered their curricula to help their students prepare for this exam. Students take Step II in the fourth year of medical school; passing it is generally a requirement to graduate. Students usually take Step III as interns during the first year after graduating from medical school. A student must pass all three exams in order to obtain a license to practice medicine.

At the onset of the clinical years, students experience a marked transition from classroom to hospital. Most schools require "core clerkships," clinical time spent in specific hospital departments. Virtually every school has clerkships in internal medicine, surgery, pediatrics, and obstetrics/gynecology. Other clerkships and electives include psychiatry, family medicine, emergency medicine, radiology, ophthalmology, otolaryngology, neurology, and anesthesiology.

The tasks and requirements for each clerkship vary, but generally students learn the basic approaches to caring for patients. Tasks include how to gather and interpret data such as vital signs, blood test results, and radiographic studies; how to examine patients and look for the signs and symptoms that indicate progression or slowing of disease states; how to write hospital progress notes, which document the care of patients and convey information to other health team members; how to "present" patients on "rounds," a formal verbal way of reporting to the medical team each morning the past events that have led a patient to his or her current state; and how to formulate a plan of care and carry it out in an efficient and effective manner.

In addition to learning how to perform the basic tasks, medical students are expected to be reading and mastering the foundations of each core clerkship. They must also become adept at the gamesmanship of rounds, which subjects student victims to "pimping"—that is, to being asked questions publicly and often accusingly—a practice designed to humiliate a student to the point that he or she will never forget the information. Students must learn, too, how to navigate from the lowest position of power—beneath attending physicians (who oversee the team), fellows (post-residency physicians in subspecialized training), medical residents and interns (post–medical school physicians-in-training), nurses, and social workers. All the while, the students must be pleasant, smart, enthusiastic, and helpful and must stand apart from other classmates sufficiently to convince everyone that they deserve an "honors" grade performance on the clerkship (equivalent to a grade of A), as opposed to "high pass" (a grade of B), "pass" (a grade of C), or "fail."

Of all the core clerkships, the most important and heavily weighted are surgery and internal medicine. Broadest in scope, they are considered to be the foundation subjects from which all other specialties and subspecialties arise. (Specialty training occurs after medical school graduation, when a graduate chooses an area of medicine on which to focus—much as a student chooses a major in college.) Both surgery and internal medicine clerkships require taking overnight "call" (working all day, throughout the night, and into the next day), and both usually require a "shelf exam," a national standardized exam run by the same organization that administers the Step tests, covering core content of the clerkship. Students always aim for high grades in these clerkships, which are largely determined by their shelf exam standardized scores.

During the end of the third year, students begin applying for internship and/or residency positions. Internships were historically focused in either internal medicine or surgery. Today, they continue as the first year of training after graduating from medical school for some specialties (such as anesthesia, radiology, neurology, dermatology, ophthalmology, and otolaryngology) before students begin their specialized residency training. Other specialty programs such as internal medicine, pediatrics, family medicine, psychiatry, and obstetrics/gynecology incorporate the internship year into their residency program.

Applying for an internship or residency is like applying for a job. Some jobs are more sought after and inspire more competition than others because of factors such as demand, location, reputation, work environment, and research opportunities. In recent years, the demand for specialty training in plastic surgery, dermatology, orthopedics, emergency medicine, and neurosurgery has been high, increasing competition for positions in these specialties. In the past, other specialties were the most competitive—for example, anesthesia was once the most difficult residency position to secure. One of the most important ways a student can increase the chances of obtaining a choice internship or residency spot is receiving honors in surgery and internal medicine clerkships.

In each year of medical school, students must cope with unique challenges and must acquire new skills, in an ever-changing, high-pressure environment. In a pre-clinical class, for example, students may have to adapt to as many as ten different lecturers for a single class and be able to decipher what each of them expects. With each new clerkship, students enter a new work environment and must constantly adapt to different personalities, working styles, assumptions and biases of colleagues, and evaluation systems. The rules seem to change daily, and students must be able to adjust instantly.

This section includes stories of students who are asking questions such as these: How am I changing now that I'm in medical school? Why am I changing? Why do I feel so different from people who aren't in medical school? Why do I feel so unsupported and alone in medical school? Do I like what I'm becoming? What kind of doctor do I want to be? Can I become the doctor I want to be? Why did I go into medicine in the first place? These questions may be even more important to a new, more diverse population of medical students, who do not as readily identify with the authority figures in their environment.

Some of the authors in Part Two make the transition to their new identities more easily (a Muslim, a young wife from a small town in Texas) than others (a man who dissociates from medical school). Others are ashamed (a "closeted" Christian), hide (a recovering alcoholic), use humor (a lesbian mother), or question the changes and sacrifices expected of them (a politically-oriented liberal arts major, a woman who also wants to play a more conventional role as wife and mother). One (a man writing about Ayurveda, the traditional medical system in India) works to integrate two different medical systems and questions the underlying assumption that Western medicine is the supreme medical model. Each writer must somehow reconcile his or her previous identity with a new professional medical identity that has traditionally imposed itself over all others.

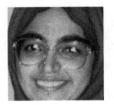

NECESSARY ACCESSORIES

M y starched white coat hung on a plastic hanger suspended from a gray steel bookshelf. Worn only once, two years ago at the White Coat Ceremony, an event that welcomed first-year students into the profession of medicine, the coat would now be used in a functional capacity for my first clinical experience. The rest of my ensemble had also been carefully prepared. My khaki pants were neatly pressed. As I admired them, I ran my fingers along their crisp creases, which rarely graced my daily wear. I left my loose-fitting, thigh-length black and beige dress shirt untucked so as not to define the shape of my body.

I took my white coat off its hanger and put it on, tugging at the stiff lapels in a vain effort to make them lie flat. The name tag above my upper left pocket read "Nusheen Ameenuddin, Student Physician." I balanced my hunter green stethoscope around my neck, letting its weight tame the intractable lapels and allowing the small golden pin embossed with the image of a heart-shaped stethoscope to be properly displayed. The pin, a gift from the medical school, symbolized compassion in medicine. I adjusted my hijab, a simple black cotton knit cloth that covered my head and neck, and tucked several stray wisps of hair underneath.

Before I left the room, I stopped for one last look in the mirror to make sure everything was right. I saw a woman who at last was able to face the public as both a medical professional and a committed Muslim. But I wondered whether others might find my appearance an unacceptable contradiction.

Without my ever saying a word, my white coat states what I do, while my hijab states who I am. Although I slipped into the white coat easily, it had taken me years to work up the courage to wear a hijab. During my junior year of high school, after years of wanting to express my religion more openly, I warned my friends that I was contemplating donning a hijab when I became a senior. When I returned to school in the fall without it, a Christian friend chastised me for failing to follow through with my commitment to my faith.

For the first few weeks of school that fall, I retained my identity as a "normal" high school student. I felt unprepared to deal with the reactions a hijab would provoke. Some might see it as interesting, even exotic, but I knew the hijab connoted "foreignness." Wearing it would make me stand out as different—intentionally different from the rest of American society. I knew that once I put it on I could no longer quietly hide Islam in my heart and choose to reveal my faith only when and to whom I wanted. To the outside world, Islam would become the accessory I wore on my head, the first and often the only thing people would see about me.

I finally decided to wear the hijab after I attended an Islamic convention. There, for an entire weekend, among other Muslims, I did not need to explain such things as why I wore long sleeves and slacks in the middle of summer (so that I did not expose my skin or appear as a sex object in public) or why I spent lunch periods in the library during the month of Ramadan (as a quiet sanctuary, it reminded me of my commitment to fasting and prayer). I did not have to worry about how to incorporate the five daily prayers into my routine. At first, I felt like a hypocrite, putting on a hijab just for the convention because I knew that it would help me to feel more a part of the group. No one would doubt my commitment to Islamic beliefs and practices. It struck me that the women around me wore their hijabs so comfortably. My first impulse was to ask the girls my age if they really wore hijabs in public and how they dealt with the negative reactions. This impulse died away as I spent more time openly acknowledging my faith among others who did the same. I no longer felt like a hypocrite or a coward. Now I resolved to live openly as a Muslim and wear my hijab in the larger community.

I returned to school wearing my hijab and waited to see what would happen. The same Christian friend who had previously chastised me now flashed me a thumbs-up. Another told me that she admired me for going against the norm. One freshman boy, who wore a Confederate flag on his backpack, teased me, calling me a "sheet head." But by the end of the year, he was chatting with me about a science project. Some people asked me about the hijab's significance, which gave me the opportunity to share a part of myself. What concerned me were the people who did not ask and who likely drew their own conclusions, accurate or not, about Islam and Muslim women. Even so, I reasoned that I had made it through the toughest time and that, beyond high school, people would be even more open, accepting, and educated.

As I became more comfortable wearing the hijab on a regular basis, I also became increasingly committed to the idea of practicing medicine. For me, words I had read in the Qur'an many times lay at the heart of what drew me to medicine: "Truly my prayer and my service of sacrifice, my life and my death are all for Allah, the Cherisher of the Worlds" (Qur'an 6:162).

Growing up, I was introduced to Islam as a peace-loving, service-oriented way of life. For Muslims, every good deed performed with the intention of pleasing God is considered worship, whether it is making a child smile, seeking knowledge, or joining the noble profession of medicine. Entering medical school was my way of fulfilling my religious duty and making my life on earth count. Like religious clerics who devote their lives to God because of a calling they feel deep in their souls, I felt a pull toward medicine and could not imagine doing anything else.

Islam also influenced my career plans because Muslims (who follow the example of the Prophet Muhammad) are exhorted to correct injustice. If we cannot take action, we must oppose injustice with speech. If speaking out is not possible, then we must feel it in our hearts. I believed that inadequate health care was an injustice that I could help to correct as a public health physician.

I was inspired by stories of my grandfather, who practiced medicine for decades in Mysore, India. Most of his patients had little money, yet he never turned anyone away from the clinic he operated out of his home. Instead, he would accept the occasional live chicken, a portion of rice, or nothing at all. In the evenings, he would check on many of his patients in their homes, often with my father or one of his five brothers in tow. For my grandfather, medicine was a service to Allah that required personal sacrifice, and I wanted to be like him.

I believed that my commitments to medicine and to Islam were inextricably linked, but I wondered whether wearing my hijab would cause others in the medical community to see a contradiction. In college, I had three advisers, two of whom warned that wearing my hijab would be a problem. They argued that growing up in a university town had sheltered me from bigotry and that citizens in some areas of our rural state were unaccepting of people who did not attend the local church. They discounted as naïve my belief that as long as I was comfortable with myself, others would accept me as a physician in their community. In fact, when I was in medical school, my hijab did at times overshadow my white coat.

Once, for example, I walked into an exam room without the benefit of an introduction from my supervising physician. When she saw me, my patient stopped in mid-sentence. Her eyes moved conspicuously from my head to my feet and then fixated on my head. Surprised by her response, I stumbled through my introduction and assured her that I was, indeed, in the right place and that I would, with her permission, be taking her medical history. She exchanged a worried look with her husband, and only after several minutes of small talk did she appear to relax.

She was not the first patient, nor would she be the last, to so obviously object to my appearance. I realized that I would have to work much harder than my classmates to put my patients at ease, and even then I might never gain their trust.

My third adviser, in contrast, encouraged me to pursue my goal of working in a rural area, while wearing a hijab. A political science professor originally from India, she suggested that I try to use my difference to establish connections within the community. Her instincts proved accurate in my experience with Mrs. Mayflower, a patient I met while I was an undergraduate student volunteering at a medical clinic in rural Kansas.

Mrs. Mayflower came into the clinic after a minor car accident. Undaunted by my hijab, she chatted with me about how important it was to her to be able to drive, in order to maintain her independence at the age of ninety-three. At the end of her visit, she patted me on the back and wished me good luck in my career.

Because of subsequent medical problems, Mrs. Mayflower came into the clinic several more times over the next few weeks. I learned that she was a lifetime resident of this small town. Every morning, she drove herself and three other elderly ladies to Mass and then volunteered as a driver for Meals on Wheels. When the doctor attempted to dissuade her from driving, she resisted, telling him, "Those people need their meals."

I came to the clinic one day to find that she had been hospitalized with severe internal bleeding in her gastrointestinal tract. I rushed to her hospital room, where I watched from a corner as the doctor and nurses worked on her. A priest performed last rites while Mrs. Mayflower's son summoned the rest of the family.

I waited for a break in the activity before approaching her bed. I leaned toward her and whispered her name. She turned toward me and her mouth opened, but no sound came out. I smiled at her, hoping she would respond, but her head rolled back on the pillow and her eyes closed. Her shallow breaths produced barely a hint of steam in her oxygen mask. Her short white hair was unkempt. Her head tilted back; her face held no trace of expression. She reminded me of the other elderly patients I had seen in the hospital, homogeneous, nameless. I was frightened. But when Mrs. Mayflower's daughter arrived, she greeted me warmly, though we had never met. "Mother told us all about you," she said.

Standing in her room with her family, as I watched what I believed were her last moments, I began a silent prayer for Mrs. Mayflower. I recited verses from the Qur'an, and I made a supplication, a *du'a*, asking God for help. But I left that night expecting that she would pass away by morning.

The next day, her doctor told me that the bleeding had stopped and that Mrs. Mayflower would live. I found her in her room, sitting up in bed eating lunch. Traces of dried blood lined her left nostril, where a plastic tube had been the night before. The pale, empty expression she had worn the previous day was gone. Now her mouth was set in a firm line as she asserted that the surgeon had no right to charge her for procedures that she had not requested. She had not lost her sense of humor.

I smiled and took her hand. "You gave us quite a scare," I told her.

"Well, I thought I was going on a trip." She paused. "You prayed for me, didn't you?"

I nodded. She knew that I had remembered her and that, despite our different religions, we turned to the same God, the One Creator. She beckoned me to lean in closer. Placing both hands on my face, she drew me in and kissed me on the cheek. "You will be a good doctor," she said.

Wearing a white coat produces a curious phenomenon. Other people seem to recognize me in a different way. After the White Coat Ceremony, as I was giving my parents a tour of the campus, a senior medical student dressed in green scrubs saw us from down the hallway. He smiled at me, and his eyes held mine for a few moments before he offered a nod of acknowledgment. The memory of his gesture stayed with me because I am not used to having people accept me so quickly, hijab and all. My white coat allows me to be instantly recognized as a member of one of the most elite societies in America.

I know that, throughout my medical career, the simple approval I get by wearing my white coat will contrast with reactions to my hijab, which can be deeper and more complicated, whether they are positive, as with Mrs. Mayflower, or negative, as with some other patients I've seen. And maybe this is how it should be, because while the white coat is just my uniform, the hijab represents my underlying reasons for putting it on.

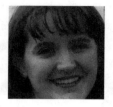

MEDICAL SCHOOL METAMORPHOSIS

L ife has changed for me in many ways since I started medical school a year ago. I study more; I play less. And I can no longer carry on a normal conversation with people outside medical school. This change seemed to occur overnight. One day I was an average twenty-three-year-old married woman from a small Texas town; the next I was a "Medical Student." This new label has changed how people look at me and how I look at the world in ways I never anticipated.

Sanger, Texas, is a typical small town of six thousand, with more churches than gas stations, where only two intersections have traffic lights. Mornings here are kicked off at the Buckhorn Café, where the same men assemble each day to drink coffee and talk about the happenings around town. Everyone at the Buckhorn knows everyone else, and all who enter the door, with its announcing jingle, are greeted by all those who arrived earlier. Life seems picturesque: our small downtown is a square surrounded by storefronts—the florist, hardware store, pharmacy, local chamber of commerce and doctor's office. Some of the old-timers can even tell you of a time when Dr. Chapman had a few rooms in his medical clinic where patients stayed overnight when they needed round-the-clock care. It's stories like these that make me want to be a doctor in a small town, where my patients can be more than a medical record number. I want my patients to be friends.

Sometimes I think about growing up in Sanger—good people, fun times, and a normal life—and I wonder why I chose to go to medical school. I was a typical high school student, whose main thought about medicine was that it would take many more years of school than I was willing to put in. A good portion of the sixty-seven students in my high school graduating class went to college, but it had been twenty years since anyone from Sanger had gone to medical school. I decided that four years of college, learning speech therapy, was the upper limit for me. Halfway through college, however, I realized that the academic work wasn't nearly as bad as I had once feared. And, by extension, I decided that maybe medical school wouldn't be as terrifying as I had heard. Deep down, I really did want to be a doctor. So I took the challenge and applied, wondering if any medical school would want a plain, small-town person like me without a background in molecular genetics or biochemical research.

To my amazement, I got in. And when I started, I discovered that there are a lot of normal and plain people here. At least, to each other we seem "normal." People looking in from the outside, however, think that only rare, exceptional people achieve the rank of Medical Student and Future Doctor. So people from my hometown, who knew me as a normal person with no mystical scientific abilities, have become incredibly curious about my experiences in medical school.

I noticed this during my first visit home. I wasn't prepared for friends and family to be so intrigued about my new life. I was overflowing with excitement about my experiences in medical school, and I longed for people to understand at least some of what I was going through—just to know what I did each day. How could I convey my experience of learning a century's worth of biochemistry in one semester? Or my amazement at anatomy dissections on a human cadaver? Or how I struggled to ask patients very personal questions while learning to take medical histories? How could I explain that I now studied more for a single test than I had ever studied during all of finals week in college? It seemed hopeless. Besides, I wanted to be treated the same as always. So I downplayed medical school and tried to talk about everyday Sanger topics: the best sale at Dillard's, Thomas and Elizabeth's wedding, the newest baby to enter the church nursery. But no matter how hard I tried, the conversation would suddenly turn.

"So, are you working on cadavers yet?"

"What's it like? How much do you study?"

"Is it really as hard as everyone says?"

Sometimes it felt as if the College of Medicine had secretly tattooed my forehead while I was sleeping: "Medical Student Freak."

But occasionally, my enthusiasm would carry me away, as it did at Mike's birthday party. I found myself describing to Aunt Betty Lou how amazing it was to look inside a human body at the perfect placement of all the organs, which fit together like a jigsaw puzzle. I told Uncle Chet about dissecting a heart—how the heart muscle looked, what the valves felt like, and how the arteries traveled around it. But I quickly realized that the average person doesn't actually enjoy descriptions of gross anatomy dissections, which I suspect are centuries-old rituals of torture that medical students are forced to endure just to prove themselves. So I managed to refrain from further details and instead ate my piece of festively decorated white birthday cake and vanilla ice cream. I evaded the rest of the questions with a canned response: "Everything is going well for us. School is great. How are you and your family doing?"

Everyone in Sanger made me feel different, and maybe a little special. Consequently, I started to change the way I thought about myself. I was no longer "normal" like them. I had crossed into a wondrous foreign realm. I was a Medical Student.

One day during my first year of medical school, I was at a family Thanksgiving gathering. I spent most of the day with various family members talking about thyroid problems, diabetes, and lumbar pain. Then my cousin sat next to me, and I offered condolences on the recent death of his father. I meant it simply as a thoughtful gesture—the sort of thing that normal people do when there's a death in the family. But then this person whom I rarely see and don't know very well spent the next half hour describing his father's death, from the diagnosis of his cancer until his final breath. He talked about medicines, details of the cancer, decisions regarding consent to surgery, and his own response to his father's death. I was honored that he seemed to find comfort in confiding in me. It was as though he automatically trusted me, simply because I'm learning to be a doctor. As I sat there listening, I suddenly realized that trust was a privilege that few are granted, and I wanted to deserve it by becoming as knowledgeable and compassionate as I could.

People often think that since I've been in medical school for a full year now, I should be able to answer all their medical questions:

"Can you bring your ear-looker to see if my ear infection is gone?"

"What's the best thing to take for hay fever?"

"What makes your stomach hurt right here?"

"Will you listen to my lungs to see if my cold has moved into my chest?"

"What's different about this new blood pressure pill?"

"Should I be on hormones?"

I have to admit that I'm sometimes afraid to answer their questions. Most of the answers I give are probably harmless, but I might tell them the wrong thing. So after every answer, I always add, "... but you should really ask your own doctor because I'm just a Medical Student." Of course, since I have little clinical experience at this point, I'm intrigued to see how my answer will compare with what their real doctor tells them. Often they're surprised by how much information I can give them. And though I'm sometimes right, that's not always the case.

In looking back over the past year, I certainly did not expect medical school to have such an impact on my life and my identity. No one told me that I would suddenly be perceived as someone who can automatically be trusted. No one told me that people expect elegant answers and magical cures from those who spend their days in a white coat with a prescription pad in the pocket. No one told me that although I am still the same person on the inside, I seem different to others simply by being a Medical Student. Although some people may see the world of medicine as confusing and distant, it's important for them to remember that doctors are still human. We are "normal" people, and some of us are from small towns in Texas.

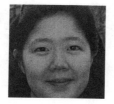

WHY AM I IN MEDICAL SCHOOL?

N o one ever said it would be easy. Nonetheless, I maintain that the past several years have been an especially difficult time in which to be a medical student. I started medical school in the fall of 1999, living in the "birthplace of Silicon Valley," as Palo Alto is known. With many of my friends from college then working for Internet start-ups, I sometimes felt jealous that they were out in a world where new and exciting ideas were changing the face of knowledge and communication (sometimes rather disturbingly), while here I was, stuck in a classroom. Once upon a time, telling a stranger that you were a medical student elicited a different, more enthusiastic response than it does these days, when the reply is usually one of pity or disinterest.

There are also people who seem to derive a perverse pleasure in telling me how doctors will be either obsolete or completely bankrupt in the next few years. My uncle, who is an electrical engineer, likes to tell me that soon, very soon, computers will be able to do anything a doctor can do, and better. My roommate, who is not a medical student, was recently visited by her family from the East Coast. When I told her mother that I was a medical student, she shook her head in pity and told me, "It's going to be a long, tough road. It's so much work, and the reward just isn't what it used to be." As if that had never occurred to me before.

Then there is the obligatory sense of personal angst—wondering whether I should have spent a year traveling the world, writing a book, or teaching in Rome. Perhaps the most difficult source of doubt about medicine for me, however, has been a vague sense that many of the concerns that originally led me to medicine are simply not valued by the medical establishment.

Since coming to medical school, I have learned that I am something of a radical. Mind you, this realization has been somewhat surprising to me, as I have never before considered my opinions particularly revolutionary. (Shulamith Firestone, Emma Goldman, and World Trade Organization protesters—now, they're what I call revolutionary.) I happen to believe that there are unacceptable disparities in health care access and treatment, and *zap!* I've turned into a communist. I express horror at the lack of sophisticated dialogue about race, or any dialogue about race that extends beyond cursory acknowledgment (although even that, at times, would be nice), and suddenly I'm one of those "political" types. I begin talking about tangible reforms in the medical curriculum, and now I'm a bona fide social activist.

Just to be clear, I never lied to the admissions committee. In case they could not gather from my major (women's studies and social anthropology), my semester abroad, my lack of published papers in *Science* or *Nature*—just in case they might have mistaken me for other than who I am—I wrote rather unequivocally in my personal statement, "I want to be a doctor because I see health as deeply politically and morally charged, and therefore full of potential for progressive change." See? I possessed no ulterior motives, no grand scheme to enter medical school as a subversive radical determined to shake up the foundations of this hallowed institution. I simply figured that if the members of the admissions committee were seeking an applicant with no interest in social medicine, government policy, cultural conflicts, gender and race politics, economic disparity, literature and art—in general, the world around me—they would not have accepted me.

Coming from an academic background in women's studies, I can assure you that I am a small fry in the world of radicalism. What is more fascinating and disturbing about my newfound radical status is precisely how *little* politicization and social consciousness it takes for someone in the medical field (even a student) to fall outside the professional mainstream. Is it important, for instance, that out of more than forty or so lecturers I have listened to, only three were women (and only one was nonwhite)? I still find it surprising that many among the faculty do not think that it is.

My undergraduate major taught me to think critically, to question the nature of power structures, to seek historical context, to ask what is at stake, and to disregard and debunk dogma (be it conservative, radical, or anything in between). Now I find myself going out on a limb merely by suggesting that perhaps we need more education and discussion around such topics as gun violence, alternative medicine, ethics in the pharmaceutical industry, and racist medical practices. As a pre-clinical student, I have listened to professors derisively dismiss all alternative and complementary medical practices as "unscientific." Such flippancy strikes me as incredibly naïve: not only does it demonstrate a total lack of historical understanding about the emergence of Western biomedicine itself, but it is also completely out of touch with the majority of Americans, let alone the rest of the world.

What I find most terrifying is the silence on even the least controversial of topics in our medical education. For me, the privilege of being a student at a university includes the rights of idealism, intellectual ferment, and independence of thought. Will I have to keep my mouth shut about wrongs I see in our profession until I am fifty years old, with the grueling hours of residency long past, and a patient base well established? Should I unlearn everything I learned in college? Deny the existence of injustice and declare fanatic belief only in Western biomedicine?

Apart from learning that I was a radical, I also came to two terribly uncharitable and not very profound conclusions during my first quarter of medical school. First, I decided that medical students were, for the most part, an unimpressive bunch. Conversations never seemed to reach beyond what I call "the med school mundane"—topics like the cranial nerves, the workload, and where to get the best coffee within a three-mile radius. Where were the future William Jameses, Anton Chekhovs, Gertrude Steins, and William Carlos Williamses (all of whom I admire and all of whom, by the way, went to medical school)? Finding myself in an environment that seems to value only basic science (concrete data, not the "fuzzy" stuff), I felt even more isolated from my peers, who seemed happy enough with what they were learning.

My second conclusion was that medical knowledge is uninteresting. In the throes of anatomy and histology, I wrote in my journal:

> I cannot get away from the nagging feeling that the people who go into medicine constitute a discrete group, and I simply do not belong. No, it's not a social exclusivity thing that makes me feel left out; it's more just that I don't feel sufficiently fascinated by the things medicine has to offer. At least as I'm learning it now. There is simply no opportunity for me to engage in the academic activities that first motivated me to go to medical school: reading, writing, discussing anything other than little dark spots, squiggly nuclei, and more goddamn anatomical relationships. Where's the context?

Hearing the rapture in the voices of certain of my classmates as they pondered bright futures as dermatologists, orthopedic surgeons, and neurosurgeons (fields that held not the slightest appeal for me), I lamented my lack of focus and felt increasing doubt in my supposed calling. "Wait, *why* am I going into medicine?" (And "How many times can I ask this each day?")

Misery, however, loves (and seeks) company; and as I became aware of the concurrent dissatisfaction of many of my classmates, I realized that my two initial judgments were closely linked and, more important, were wrong. When I spoke with students more intimately, I realized that there were others like me. It simply took time for us to identify one another.

As pre-clinical students, we never have any forums in which we can learn about each other and the incredible wealth of experiences and accomplishments that we collectively bring to medical school. We have virtually no class time devoted to discussing the whole slew of motivations that brought us into medicine: belief (at least to some degree) in the biomedical model; a desire to combat poverty, disease, and racial disparities in care; a search for prestige or financial stability; personal experiences of prejudice and discrimination; commitment to our communities. With thirty hours a week of class time spent sitting in a lecture hall looking at PowerPoint slides, who has the time? As the workload and stress mount, discussion of anything outside the required basics becomes superfluous, unimportant, and an added headache. Virtually no one wants to attend a voluntary two-hour symposium on the ethics of transplanting embryonic tissue into the brains of Parkinson's patients—after all, who wants to spend extra time and energy caring about stuff we aren't tested on?

With all these difficulties, why, indeed, am I in medical school? When I was in high school, I stopped going to church because I disagreed with what I perceived to be a sexist statement in the preacher's sermon. (He asserted that our country's high unemployment rate was a result of the large numbers of women who had entered the workforce following the women's liberation movement.) I was also perilously close to losing my faith. My father then gave me a guiding piece of advice. He told me that there may be problems with an institution and particular individuals, but they do not constitute, nor should they obscure, what I believe to be good and right.

Despite all my righteous anger at faulty structures in the health care system and the medical curriculum, I maintain my belief in the underlying nobility of the medical profession and its potential to effect profound and positive social change. It has been difficult for me to work within such a flawed system of medical training while at the same time maintaining my broader perspective. I hope, however, that I can stick with it, that my colleagues will continue to amaze and sustain me, that my clinical judgments will not become obsolete in five years (!), and that I will always be challenged and stimulated by what this profession can offer. Most important, I never want to lose my idealism about what medicine can and should be.

MY SECRET LIFE

My name is Linda, and I am a third-year medical student at a well-respected medical school in New York. I am also an alcoholic. You would never know that by looking at me. I am a student in good standing, comport myself in a professional manner, get along well with my colleagues, and do not embarrass myself at class functions. My path to medical school, however, has been different from that of most of my classmates. That path has most recently been laid, brick by brick, by the fellowship of Alcoholics Anonymous, but it began with my first drink.

Many young people enjoy drinking and partying and may even go through a phase of heavy drinking in high school or college. But my drinking was different. I began drinking when I was thirteen years old, not to have fun but to escape the pain of living inside my own skin. At that time, I didn't know why I was drinking; I knew only that I felt different from everyone else. But alcohol changed all that. With a few drinks in me, I suddenly felt cool, witty, and gorgeous; my clothes were no longer out of style, my acne disappeared, and I magically lost twenty-five pounds. If drinking had negative consequences, I didn't care. What alcohol did for me made whatever consequences it brought worth the price, at least until toward the end of my drinking career.

As years passed, my schoolwork began to suffer, as did my relationship with my family. I paid attention to alcohol and little else. Though I had wanted to be a doctor, alcohol became more important. I dropped out of the private high school I had been attending on a scholarship and graduated to a barstool. Within a week, I found myself handcuffed in the back of a police car after driving around for hours in a blackout. After that, I curtailed my driving but not my drinking; giving up alcohol was simply not an option.

I drank at every opportunity, finding ways to get alcohol as a minor. For example, I would frequent sleazy little beer bars that weren't particular about checking IDs. I gravitated instinctively to such places, bars where older men and hard-bitten women sat twirling their beer glasses. Paroled felons from Folsom Prison congregated at one of my favorite haunts. One could obtain an unregistered gun there, and the former bartender had recently been shot and killed. Little did I care, as a clueless eighteen-year-old suburban girl, that I placed my life in danger every time I set foot in there. All I knew was that they charged thirty-five cents for a glass of draft beer and never checked my ID. What more did I need to know?

I also got alcohol at the local convenience store, where I would ask the unsavory characters hanging around outside to buy me a bottle. I had money, they had legal IDs, so we were instant friends. We'd sit in the weeds behind the store after midnight and drink, me and the homeless men twice my age. One of them chased me home one night and tried to rape me, but I managed to get rid of him—and I'd gotten my liquor, so I didn't much care. Other times, I'd party with the hippie-intellectual-artist types. Things got wild, with loud rock bands and flowing kegs. Often the party would end in a soddenly ineffectual orgy. But other nights, many nights, I drank alone.

At age twenty, I moved in with an unemployed man in his forties. He didn't work, and I barely hung on to my own menial job. I made two hundred dollars a week and paid one hundred sixty-five dollars a month for rent; the rest of the money went to alcohol. Our curtains were a blanket tacked over the window, our living room furniture was made of milk crates I stole from work, and our bed was a foam rubber mattress that we found in the street. Before long, I was living alone again.

One day, the unthinkable happened—alcohol quit working for me. No matter how much I drank, my glamorous delusions were replaced by a queasy anxiety that wouldn't go away. Desperate to feel better, I tried unsuccessfully to stop drinking. I couldn't eat, sleep, or think. My thinking degenerated—I had a brain tumor, I was going to get food poisoning, "they" were coming to get me. Somehow I still managed to show up for work, because I needed money for my liquor. But I knew it was only a matter of time before I would hole up with a bottle until my money ran out. I couldn't imagine life either with alcohol or without it, and I wished only for the end. I was just twenty-one years old.

·   ·   ·   ·   ·

No one gets to their first AA meeting when they're on a winning streak. At my first meeting, I could barely construct a coherent sentence. My sponsor and other AA members taught me how to rebuild my life, one day at a time. Using the Twelve Steps, I got through a day, then a week, and then a month and more, without drinking.

After eighteen months of sobriety in AA, I suffered a major depression that eventually led me to a new life. Unable to work, I checked myself into an alcohol recovery house. During that time, I realized that, to recover, I had to do more than recite the Twelve Steps; I had to embrace them as a lifestyle. In doing so, I gained an awareness of a loving God who had entered my heart and would always guide me through any ongoing recovery. Though I'd like to say that I never again thought about suicide or taking a drink, I can't. But I now had an inner resource.

My depression started to lift, and I went to vocational counseling. Deep down, I wanted to be a doctor, but I thought that was impossible now. I was a high school dropout alcoholic, emerging from a crippling depression, who hadn't worked in fourteen months. Instead, I trained to work as a medical secretary. The night before I began my new job as a medical records clerk, I lay awake for hours, certain that they had mixed up the applications and hired me by mistake. Tomorrow, surely, they would find out that I really wasn't good enough to do a nice, clean job that would let me use my mind.

Despite my fears, I did a fine job. After working there a few months, I began to wonder if I could possibly go to college. I signed up for two night courses that went well, and I decided to go to school full time during the day. I cut back my work hours, took out a loan, and became a real student. I wanted to take pre-med courses, but, because medical school seemed so improbable, I majored in humanities instead. When I graduated with my associate's degree, I was stunned to find out that I had been chosen valedictorian. This honor gave me the courage to transfer to the local state university to finish my bachelor's degree.

While completing my degree, I went through counseling and remembered that my father had sexually abused me when I was three years old. The tenets of AA helped me work through all the pain, grief, terror, and rage that I had unknowingly carried inside and that drinking had allowed me to forget. Somehow I managed to stay sober, forgave my father, and finished my degree.

After graduation, while working as an administrative assistant for a medical research group, my desire to become a doctor was rekindled. As I sat across from the principal scientist, it occurred to me that I wanted to do what he did—interesting and challenging work—rather than what I did, which was boring and safe. For the first time, I recognized my desire for what it was—a calling, a passion, my own true destiny. I could not turn my back on it without stifling my spirit. I was afraid that if I did that, I would someday drink again.

. . . . .

Within a year, I returned to school to undertake my prerequisite science courses. When I finally dropped my medical school application in the mail, I realized that I stood a good chance of getting in. I didn't know whether to be thrilled or terrified.

Once in medical school, I had to face some new realities. I knew that I had to establish a connection with AA as soon as possible, since I was in a new city without a support group; but this proved difficult, given my hectic class schedule. I went to as many meetings as I could, but fewer than I had been accustomed to attending. Although it was harder to stay sober, I managed; I wasn't about to let go of my dream.

The more difficult problem, however, was that for the first time it was critical to keep my AA membership secret. The medical profession mostly takes a dim view of alcoholism. Alcoholics are those despicable patients who show up in the emergency room at inconvenient times, with only themselves and their weak wills to blame for their problems. Doctors can't be alcoholics; if a doctor with a drinking problem is found out, he or she is often subjected to both formal and informal censure. Of course, the quality of patient care and safety should always be the primary concern, but I think that the medical culture is intolerant of weakness in its members and is therefore unsympathetic.

A man I knew in AA went through medical school and residency in recovery. When he applied for licensure, he truthfully answered the application question about his past treatment for alcoholism. Despite sixteen years of sobriety and his stellar clinical performance, he was required to register as an "impaired physician." He regretted his honesty. Another man I met in AA was a former medical student who had been suspended for academic failure as a result of his drinking. He, too, had been honest with the school's administration and explained what he was doing to achieve sobriety. He was denied readmission even after two years of sobriety. The last I heard he was still sober, attending medical school in the Caribbean. These stories confirmed my intuition that it would be wise to keep my alcoholism and AA membership secret. AA requires "rigorous honesty," but not when that would unfairly ruin one's life. So whenever the medical school health forms screen for alcohol use, I answer "no" with a clear conscience.

I had believed that keeping my AA membership secret would be simple. But it isn't that easy. Never have I so carefully guarded my anonymity. For example, one of the mandatory core clerkships, psychiatry, requires its students to attend an AA meeting, so there's always a chance of running into another medical student there. I could pretend to be just another observer—unless I happen to be chairing the meeting that night. Sometimes I'll peer into the window before I go into an AA meeting, to make sure no one from my medical school is there. Then I go in, relieved, if only for this time. Other times, to avoid the fear of trying to hide, it seems easier to drive far out of town to attend a meeting.

I worry about my classmates, but it's also possible that my supervising physicians, course director, or dean could find me out. Whether or not discovery becomes a problem for me depends on the person's attitude toward alcoholism, experience with alcoholics, and power to affect my career. For instance, any mention of alcoholism could jeopardize my post–medical school residency application. I just can't take the chance of being open and honest about being an alcoholic, even though I've been sober for seventeen years.

Sneaking into AA meetings may be a small price to pay for staying sober in medical school. For me, the larger issue is that the medical establishment could see my AA membership as a liability. In AA, I have faced myself, found a new way to live, and developed compassion for my own suffering and that of others. I have spent the past seventeen years sharing my innermost thoughts and feelings with AA members of every race, age, gender, and social class. I have sat in meetings with a corporate executive on my right and a paranoid schizophrenic on my left, all of us there for the same reason. I have held a sobbing man in my arms to comfort him, without even knowing his name. I have discovered how vulnerable we all are, how fragile, how precious. How does any of this render me unfit or unworthy to be a doctor?

I believe that we need more doctors who understand alcoholism and recovery. The contempt alcoholics receive from some doctors only compounds the shame, guilt, and isolation of alcoholism. As a medical student, I can't always challenge the way an alcoholic is being treated by the medical team, but I can show the patient my own compassion. And sometimes I have the chance to talk to an alcoholic patient, to let him or her know there is another way to live.

. . . . .

Despite the pressures of medical school, I remain active in AA. I don't believe medical school is more difficult for sober alcoholics than it is for anyone else. In some ways, it might be easier. With everything I've been through, the opportunity to do work I love is a gift, not a burden. I still attend meetings, stay in contact with my sponsor, and sponsor others. I believe that out of my experience as an alcoholic comes the potential to be a better doctor. This is my secret life.

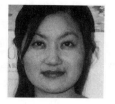

FIVE POINTS OFF FOR GOING
TO MEDICAL SCHOOL

Seeing the bare trees braced against the chilly November wind, I
think of the freezing cold winter that is fast approaching. This will
be my second winter in New York, far away from my home in California. After living most of my life with relatively mild transitions
between seasons, I must remind myself why I am here.

For most of my classmates, getting into medical school may have
been the greatest accomplishment of their lives to this point, their
crowning scholastic victory over a lifetime of educational pressures and
demands. I, on the other hand, have some ambivalence about being in
medical school. Others may share some of my issues, but none of my
classmates are Christian Korean women in the navy, like me.

I grew up in a traditional Korean household, where all the girls
played the piano and covered their mouths when they laughed. I was
constantly reminded that no matter how rich or famous I became, my
happiness would never be complete without the "right man" and a family. The most important purpose in my life was to "marry well." When
I decided to go to the University of California at Berkeley for college,
most people thought, "Good, she can get her 'MRS' degree and find
herself a successful husband."

Before Berkeley, I had always thought that was my future—marriage, family, and making a home. That was my mother's life, and I appreciated the warm meals, fresh laundry, and words of encouragement that she provided in abundance at home. My mother treated my father with utmost respect, spoke to him in the "honorific" form in Korean, and always served him first. She played the supporting role when it came to his work as a pastor and took care of any family business that might have distracted him from it. In those days, I could only see myself growing up to be just like her.

At Berkeley, the world became larger and more complicated. Suddenly, a college graduate of twenty-one or twenty-two (considered marrying age in Korean culture) didn't seem so old anymore, especially given that many of the guys I met seemed too immature even to consider marriage. I discovered a dichotomy between what I once thought was my future and my ambition to attain the American Dream, in which I could be anything I wanted. But just because I could, did that mean I should? I was completely clueless as to what I wanted to do with the rest of my life.

When I decided to go into medicine, few people approved. My parents were proud of me but felt torn between wanting me to have a successful career and wanting me to "settle down." They were nervous because my focus was on being a pre-med student at a time when they believed that a woman should be thinking about marriage and family. On the pre-med track, I was caught up in the race: getting points for volunteer work, research, letters of recommendation, and grades.

It wasn't until my junior and senior years that I seriously contemplated my future. Although I enjoyed my life and studies in the liberal world of Berkeley, I was left with too many choices, no role models, and the guilt of considering the anti-feminist and ethnocentric role of a Korean housewife. My dreams of domestic tranquility were no longer so sweet and simple.

As graduation approached, I took a weekend to fast and pray. That weekend, I sensed that God's will directed me to apply to medical school. Soon after, I received my acceptance letter to New York Medical College.

Although many expressed admiration and enthusiasm, one of my closest friends, a traditional Korean man, said, "Five points off for getting into med school." He explained that I would have difficulty finding a Korean man who would want to marry a Korean woman who was "too smart" or too busy to have dinner ready every night, let alone have *his* children. I thought my friend was being a bit extreme, but I figured that there would be plenty of professional Korean men who would not feel threatened by a woman in medicine.

Realizing that medical school would be quite costly, I looked into many options and found that the military offered a scholarship that would cover all my expenses. Although it involved a big commitment, having an enormous debt seemed more of a commitment, so I decided to apply. Pleased when I found out that I had been awarded the scholarship, I called that same friend and shared my good news. His immediate response was, "That one is ten points off!" I hadn't considered that being a doctor and a navy officer might be even more threatening.

I was disappointed that my friend didn't share my enthusiasm, but his sentiments are the same as those I face each time I go home. I am bombarded by my parents' friends questioning my choice to go to medical school. Am I dating? Why do I want to study more? Wasn't college enough? Have I met any potential doctor-husbands? How old am I again? How many more years left? I see grim expressions, faces etched with worry, voices sympathetic with pity. Is it that dismal and hopeless?

Coming to medical school, I find myself constantly in a state of conflict. I have always had a deep desire to belong to a community where family values mean everything and where there is harmony across the generations. As a Korean, I identify with the traditional roles within the family and society. As a Christian, I desire to be the type of woman described in the Bible in Proverbs 31:10–12, "a wife of noble character." On the other hand, I believe that I was called here for a purpose; getting into medical school could not be mere chance. It must be part of God's plan for me. But when I go to the mall or to church, I sometimes feel a heaviness in my heart as I watch what "normal" people do.

I have come to realize that medical school is simultaneously all about sacrifice and investment. Unlike students in most other countries, who start medical school in college, we begin after college in the United States. That is four years of college, plus four years of medical school, and at least three years of residency. I will be giving up my prime child-bearing years to study medicine. (I can't help but laugh a little at how sad but funny this sounds.) After taking classes about all the things that can go wrong with pregnancy, it's hard not to think about my aging oocytes and the statistics showing the likelihood of genetic abnormalities with increased maternal age. Nothing can stop it or slow it down. It doesn't help any that my mother calls regularly to remind me that my biological clock is ticking. And it doesn't help that some of my friends are getting engaged, and some have recently married.

As a doctor, I will make a comfortable living. Some will admire me for being a physician and a navy officer. But no amount of money or prestige can buy the family life of which I have always dreamed, complete with family dinners, storytelling at bedtime, greeting my kids after school, pets, and the PTA. I wish I could live vicariously through the experiences of my friends and family who chose the "other path," but I cannot. And yet, I see very few women doctors excelling in both medicine and family life, and even fewer that I would want as role models. Then again, there are many bright women who sacrifice career for husband and family. Do they ever wonder and regret?

Overdramatic? Probably. Unreasonable? I don't think so. Whether we like it or not, we live in a society of point systems. There are different standards, and some things are worth more or less depending on who is keeping count. Points are added or subtracted based on many things: appearance, personality, career, religion, connections. For some people, I may have gained points; yet in my world, I have lost fifteen points for the choices I have made. I wonder if there is any way to earn them back. Someone once wrote, "To choose to do something is to choose not to do a thousand other things." I've come to the realization that life choices are all about time, and I do not consider myself young anymore.

I can't predict how my perspective will change over time. My life paradigm has shifted compared to even five years ago, when I started college. How much more will I change by age thirty? Age fifty? Will it become an unbearable contradiction to serve in the U.S. military, which once was at war with Korea and threatened the very existence of the traditions I have so valued? Will I find that I cannot go back to being a traditional Korean wife and mother, even if I give up medicine? Could I ever give up medicine? I can state with certainty that I have begun to love medicine, and I cannot imagine ever trading this experience for anything or anyone. The challenges, the silent victories, the intense reality that the small things I do might make big differences in the lives of others are what keep me going.

As a devoted Christian, I should assume that God will show me the way. Yet I can't help but sigh whenever I pass by a baby in a stroller. But just as the desolate winter trees will again be covered by the blossoms of spring, I may turn a corner again and find that God has set me on a path that somehow provides all the rewards I need.

KEVIN M. TAKAKUWA

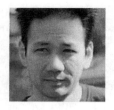

PARASYMPATHIZING

I 'm suspended in Jeanine's brown sofa, enveloped in soft velour that caresses my arms and legs. Through the windows, I can see flowering dogwood tree branches reaching toward me, inviting me outside onto the old Washington, D.C., cobblestone streets to pay witness. I sleepily imagine stuffy statesmen wearing white pony-tailed wigs and tight-fitting, gray-tailed suits, stepping over or averting their eyes from the slaves sleeping beneath the pink arms of the dogwood. But I'm not tempted to move. Not now. Just below the window sits Jeanine, propped up, facing me, mirroring my position. She speaks softly, slowly, holding me with her voice.

We've been talking for an hour now, continuing one of our many conversations from three years ago, when we were roommates on the other coast. We met serendipitously through a housing ad and ended up sharing a large two-bedroom townhouse, a modern suburban home with a dishwasher, laundry room, and "central AC," the first time I had lived with such modern conveniences. But despite the 100-degree weather, I couldn't bring myself to pay for the air conditioner, so I would always turn it off after Jeanine had turned it on. It became one of our running jokes. It was during our time in that house that Jeanine came to know the beginnings of my medical school years.

. . . . .

Ideally, I thought, medical school was about mastering basic medical principles, learning to monitor life with specialized sensors placed cleverly into the heart, and memorizing medications and doses for high blood pressure and diabetes. After all, prescribing too little or too much insulin might lead to catastrophe. We would learn, in some cases, how to override a defective body response in order to maintain life.

Grant, a new classmate who was bicycling off campus with me during our first month of school, spoke with shameless optimism about the powers of medicine and described medical school as a "privilege" that granted us the ability to indulge in academic pursuits without being bothered by the same day-to-day worries as others—like getting a job or earning a real living. Images flashed at me: consoling a close college friend who had just seroconverted to HIV-positive; then, several years later, standing over his ravaged, lifeless body. I turned my attention back to Grant. He continued on about how our minds would be spared these annoyances so that we could focus on the important "intellectual" challenge ahead. I wondered what happy drug he was taking.

Though I wanted to share Grant's idealized view of medical school, I couldn't. I had to learn how to medically care for the members of my community, one that was suffering, dying, and grieving. It had become my mission. I knew that I was able. In spite of my background in business, I believed that I could make it through medical school by hard work and persistence, the same traits that had enabled me to endure the prerequisite basic science courses during a time when my peers were establishing their careers, buying houses, settling down, having babies, and dying.

I barely scraped by in the new, arcane realm of the hard sciences, earning grades that got me into medical school but knowing that I had no conceptual understanding of what I was studying and certainly no level of mastery. I knew that I would start at a disadvantage and have to perform at the same level as the majority, who had studied science for the past four years. But I convinced myself that medicine was the best path for me because it was the most significant way to try to ensure the survival of my community—and myself.

In medical school, classes seemed to last a lifetime, hours piled on hours, information haphazardly spewed at us, disorganized and incoherent. I sat there, helpless, continuously assaulted with more and more data, quietly hoping that something, anything, was sticking to my overtaxed memory banks. Lectures began at 8:00 A.M. and consisted of back-to-back one- to two-hour blocks until noon, with ten-minute breaks between classes. But lectures ran over, with each lecturer blaming the preceding one for cutting into class time, emphasizing the need to get through the material in order to prepare us "for the test."

These key words reinforced our fear of failing and pressured us to forego our breaks. Tests became the focus of our education—we had to answer at least 70 percent of the questions correctly. We succumbed to the lecturers' threats, afraid to miss any class and too scared to protest openly. Tests, we were reminded frequently, were drawn from anything that had ever been said in our lecture or written in the course reading syllabus, the laboratory manual, or textbooks so large that they were cut in half so they could be transported more easily.

During lunch, a few students would frolic in the central courtyard playing Frisbee or hackysack. Many retreated to the lab rooms to prepare for afternoon lectures and labs or to practice answering test questions on the school's computers. I usually tried to escape the suffocating environment temporarily, hoping to find refuge from the assault of information.

One day, I stopped to collect my school mail before my escape. In the core of the block of mailboxes, where the administrative assistants stood to sort our mail, I spotted a classmate through my mailbox vista. She was huddled on the ground, chin on her knees and arms hugging her legs, crying in silence. I knew that she had lost control in the pace of school. I wanted to reassure her that "everything would work out," give her the day off, bring her hot cocoa, and tuck her into bed, but I shared her sentiments and wouldn't have accepted any reassuring words myself. Who was I to her, anyway, but another face in the crowd? For now, recognizing that she was at least safe, I gave her the only thing I thought she would allow—her privacy.

After our hour lunch break, we reconvened for four more hours of lab and/or lectures. By the end of the day, I felt like a paper towel dumped in a torrid river of knowledge, expected to stop the flow by absorbing the current. Any flicker of remaining energy I had was instinctively shunted to my motor system—to get me home immediately. I couldn't form coherent sentences, and I lost all ability to function socially.

After a quick dinner at home, I had at most four hours left for studying each night (allowing for sleep and showers), hours that were available only if I neglected grocery shopping, housecleaning, cooking, laundry, bill paying, and maintaining any outside human contact. I had been told that for every hour of lecture, I should be studying three hours at home. Based on my calculations, there weren't enough hours in the week to do this and sleep. I tried repeatedly to make do with less sleep, but I found that the next day I couldn't learn, stay awake, or feel human. And when I pushed myself to finish reading another chapter of physiology, to memorize just one more step of the Krebs cycle, my body would shut down my ambitious but overwhelmed brain, and I would awaken the next morning sprawled across my kitchen table, my books rippled with streaks of saliva.

With each passing day, I managed only to accumulate more uncompleted assignments and tasks. Days started running into one another, weeks lost meaning, seasons never seemed to change. When I was in contact with others outside the medical school, I stared at them, unable to recognize any similarities between us. The only reference points I had in time and to people were punctuated by our exam schedule.

The rest of the class appeared happy. People would stand in groups smiling at each other, trying to seem at ease, and jockeying to speak the loudest, to be the funniest, or to boast the most about *not* studying. (I later discovered that despite the public protestations, in private virtually everyone studied intensely.) The topics of their conversations never went beyond the lectures, upcoming tests, or current television shows. I never heard one criticism about our program's method of education. Yet privately I had learned that large numbers were taking Prozac to cope, that many were insecure about making it through med school, and that some were struggling in their marriages and personal relationships.

Everyone but me seemed to know the rules of appropriate topics. When I tried to talk about the lack of available tutors, the school's dismissal policies, the possibility of converting from an inherently competitive grading system to a pass/no pass system, or improving the curriculum and teaching, I was ignored, discounted, or attacked. I was seen as a troublemaker. When I patiently consoled a classmate who was having marital problems, she stopped speaking to me after she reconciled with her husband. When I tried to talk with a learning-disabled student who was struggling to pass classes, he denied that he had a learning disability. And when I told a classmate about a dean who was offering preferential treatment to white students, he replied, "It's a good thing that I'm white, then."

Many of my fellow students had no qualms about stepping on others to get to the top of the heap. "Gunners," as they were euphemistically called (referring to people who shot down others), bragged openly about getting the highest test score. They asked loudly, while in groups, how anyone could have done poorly on such an "easy" exam, when the class grading report clearly showed that some had failed. They hid important exam information from others. They faked illnesses during exams to gain more study time and to ask others which test questions had been used. I was dumbfounded. We were adults, in medical school, preparing for a profession regarded for its service to others and its high ethical standards. I couldn't believe the tactics that were employed to get the highest score, achieve a high class rank, or be voted into the honor society. Though we had been forced to compete to gain acceptance into med school, we had all made it. The game was over, the competition irrelevant. We had to learn to work collaboratively from now on.

Eventually, it became obvious that most of my classmates had built large walls around themselves. And though they may have felt safe within their walls, I could only question their poor coping skills. Why had they chosen to attend medical school? What would happen when they graduated? Would they be patient advocates? Or were they in it only to make money, gain prestige, and follow in their family's footsteps? I didn't expect everyone to have values similar to mine, but I did expect that some individuals would. Fortunately, I had a few close friends, but our time constraints, combined with their commitments to significant others, left me alone most of the time.

My convictions and morals began to haunt me. I refused to study old exams, a practice I believed was unethical and counterproductive to real understanding. I wanted to learn conceptually, to know the purpose behind the information. But there was no time for this, and there was no efficient way for me to grasp the material. I tried to adapt, altering my strategies iteration after iteration, but to no avail. Every quarter, I struggled to pass. Sometimes I hovered around the class mean, but other times I fell to the lower end of the grading curve. As the quarters ground on, I couldn't avoid hearing the gossip that separated people into categories: smart or dumb.

Daisy, in charge of tutoring services, was plainly visible through her office window facing our central courtyard. She sat motionless for hours playing computer solitaire, moving one stack of cards to the next, back and forth, black on red, red on black, ace-two-three. When I rapped on her door, she jumped.

"Oh, yes, uh, hold on a second. What can I do for you?" she asked as she scrambled to change computer screens.

"I need help with biochemistry."

"Oh, okay. I'll get you a tutor right away. When do you want to start?" Her voice dripped saccharine.

"As soon as possible. How about tomorrow?"

"I'll let you know right away."

"Thanks, Daisy. I'm desperate. I don't get biochemistry. I did terrible on my midterm and have to pass."

"Don't worry. You'll be fine. You just have to work a little harder. I'm on it right away. Just let me know if there's anything else I can do for you."

"Thanks, I'll wait to hear from you."

As I turned to leave, she turned back to solitaire. Every day when I returned, she was startled out of her game, and we replayed the same routine as if I had never spoken to her before. After a couple of weeks of playing Groundhog Day, and getting nearer to the final exam, I gave up and made an appointment with the dean. He referred me back to Daisy. "I assure you she will get you help," he asserted as he led me out of his office.

Eventually, I failed two classes: pathology and biochemistry. Though I had been struggling, I had managed to pass my classes for an entire year and thus was unaccustomed to failure. Of five thousand applicants, only ninety-three of us had made it this far. With so many applicants to choose from, I reasoned, the admissions committee must have thought that I could do this. So what could I do to succeed?

I was notified a day before the pathology retake that I hadn't passed the original exam, that I had accumulated 748 out of 1,000 possible points, two short of passing. Because of conflicting obligations, I wasn't allowed to sit for the retake exam. As for biochemistry, I had the lowest class score, one exam question away from an F and three away from a C. For that, I was allowed to sit for the retake exam, scheduled for the third day of the next quarter. If I didn't pass it, I would be placed on academic probation and my next failure would likely lead to dismissal.

That long winter break, I pored over biochemical minutiae for ten to twelve hours a day, seven days a week, for three straight weeks, fearing that my failure to memorize every fact ever mentioned in decades of biochemical research would end my medical school career. Proline, valine, arginine. How to construct an amino acid sequence, given the different rules for enzymatic cleavage. I saw no connection between the abstraction of amino acid structures and the experience of clinical medicine. But I pressed on, convincing myself that the end justified the means.

When my classmates returned, fresh from winter break, no one knew what I had endured. I had spent the holiday sequestered from the world, secluded in what felt like a biochemical prison. During study breaks, I replayed in my mind what had gone wrong and wondered why I had been sentenced, especially since I knew that biochemistry had eluded others, too, who had been saved only by the narrow whim of a grading curve. I had planned not to reveal my humiliating failure to anyone. But I had not spoken to anyone in three weeks, and the first two classmates I met heard a manic, bulimic recollection of events. Both of them paused, looked at me oddly, offered trite condolences, then scurried off.

My hope of breaking through the walls my classmates had constructed was smashed. My peers in my former life had believed that collectively we could change the world, that we needed to support one another, that there was room for us all to succeed together, and that one's success didn't depend on another's failure. But no one here was going to listen to me and offer words of comfort. No one here was going to offer to tutor me should I fail again. No one here was going to organize a protest against biochemistry, the poor teaching of the class, or the unfair grading curve, even though most hated the class and complained about the obscure test questions. I would never experience synergistic working relationships with others in medical school.

Half a year later, I experienced a third failure, this time in pharmacology. Now as I walked through the hallways, my eyes did not engage others. I was as foreign to those around me as an insomniac's sleep at midnight. Rage, despair, and disappointment, in combinations previously unknown to me, grew inside me but remained tightly reined in and escaped only when I left them unguarded.

Fortunately, I did have support at home for one year. When I passed my pharmacology retake, Jeanine posted a colorful handmade sign on my bedroom door exclaiming, "Congratulations! I knew you could do it. You're awesome!" And when I failed my biochemistry retake, one that a medical student with a Ph.D. in biochemistry barely passed, she consoled me with Ben and Jerry's ice cream. And when I made up for my two missing points in pathology by spending 160 hours of my "free time" doing a pet project for the professor, Jeanine sat with me, listened to my outrage, and calmed me down. At the end of the year, Jeanine moved to the East Coast, and I moved into my clinical years.

.   .   .   .   .

Sitting in Jeanine's Washington, D.C., apartment, she and I continue to talk, just nine hours after my journey across the country on my first real break from school in three years. I notice my lower back relaxing just enough to make contact with the sofa. As my eyes drift closed, I catch an unfamiliar awkward moment. Jeanine suddenly looks at me, differently. "Where are you living now?" she mouths, just loud enough for me to hear.

My eyes snap open. For an instant, time moves as slowly as the leak of air passing through my lips. I've only casually and selectively alluded to my living situation, not sure that anyone would understand it. But I remember from our many late nights spent discussing politics and social structures, and uncloseting our ghosts, that I don't need to be guarded around Jeanine. I'm safe in her haven, thousands of miles away from my life as a fourth-year med student still on the brink of dismissal. I've never completed the story to anyone, or organized it, or fully understood it myself. I haven't had the time to consider it. But it feels right now, finally, and I know that somehow I must explain it.

.   .   .   .   .

A fourth and then a fifth failure hit early during my first clinical year, both by the slimmest of margins, and I was ready to leave rather than face dismissal once again. After all, no one would notice my departure. My professors, who stood in front of the ninety-three of us every day or two and lectured out toward largely overwhelmed and sleep-deprived students, certainly wouldn't take note of a missing face. The administrators and deans wouldn't pay attention unless an F grade appeared on the final grading roster at the end of a term. Besides one or two friends, no one else would notice, unless it made for good gossip. When a student was dismissed, stories quickly circulated:

"Sue got kicked out of school. She totally deserved it."

"I knew Sue was cheating on that test—she kept looking over in my direction and going to the bathroom during our final."

"She told Mark that she was leaving for medical reasons."

"Sue never studied; she's so lazy."

"Well, it was obvious to me from the start that Sue wasn't cut out to be a doctor..."

Once a student was placed on academic probation, control over scheduling classes or developing a working plan to rectify any deficiencies was stripped away by the administrators, who believed in some paternalistic way that they were "helping." At least, that's what they told me during my academic probation hearing. In that narrow rectangular room, flanked by seven professors and two deans who sat speechless, staring at me, I knew exactly what they expected of me. When asked leading questions by the head of the committee, I had to humbly admit my failings, accept responsibility for those failings, and outline what I would do to avoid failing again, which meant taking time off to study after I finished my current clinical duties. I couldn't show any emotion except for deep regret, and at the end of the hearing I had to thank them for the opportunity to repent. Any deviation from this pattern would lead to serious repercussions; it already had for some individuals I knew. I can't remember what else they said during the five-minute meeting, but by the end of it I had shredded my notice into thirty-two equal pieces under the conference table.

That was the day I stopped caring about medical school, and I knew that I couldn't maintain my current life anymore. Something had to change. I was caught between a desperate urge to escape and a stubborn refusal to quit.

My decision wasn't planned, nor was it rational; but it seemed like a natural and instinctive transition. I gave up my apartment near the medical center and moved all my belongings into storage. For the first time in a while, I felt relief, as if I had gained some distance from the place that had so many acrid associations. I thought I was prepared to deal with the consequences of what I was about to do. If I failed my makeup exam and were dismissed (a strong possibility) or if I finally reached my limit and quit (another likely possibility), I could quickly pull out of town. Until then, I would return to school only when absolutely necessary and get out as fast as possible. This shortsighted plan seemed to be my best option for survival. The next week, early Monday morning, I threw two weeks of supplies into my small pickup truck, enough to get me close to finishing my current clinical course, and returned to school.

.   .   .   .   .

It was midnight. I figured that most people in this tiny town would be sleeping by now. I drove around the streets, crisscrossing through central Davis, searching for something I had never sought, not knowing if it existed. Too light there. Too secluded there. Too many cars on one street, too few on another. This neighborhood, where I once lived at the Orange Tree Apartments, named for the twin orange trees holding sour, out-of-reach fruits that marked the entrance, seemed oddly unfamiliar. Too many pedestrians there. Too close to the police station there.

I gripped the steering wheel a bit tighter. My sleepy anxiety became quiet desperation. I noticed that my odometer registered eight miles now, all driven within a one-mile grid, and I contemplated the gallon of wasted gas, a cost I couldn't afford every night. Self-conscious, I glanced around again. Had anyone noticed me? Was I driving suspiciously? I couldn't look forever, so I narrowed down my choices.

I finally settled on a street with relatively few houses, across from an elementary school. It was 1:15 A.M. now, and I struggled to remain awake. I parked between two houses so that either neighbor would attribute my truck to the other. Strangely, I had not considered the logistics of my current situation until now. I had no bathroom, so I sheepishly relieved myself on a nearby tree, which belonged to one of the $375,000 houses. I had no water to brush my teeth; I couldn't wash my hands or face. My contact lenses stuck to my eyelids. The passenger seat of my truck contained assorted medical texts, duffel bags stuffed with green scrubs, plastic bags filled with the leftover focaccia bread and fig bars that had been my dinner, and cotton shirts, pants, and silk ties that lay near the hangers that had once kept them fresh. My belongings melded together in one heaped mass.

I struggled to find comfort. In the driver's seat, I could barely move my legs. Confined, restricted, wanting to stretch across my queen-sized bed, now in storage, I failed to understand what had become of my life. I thought about everything I had exchanged for medical school: my community, my old friends, my free time, and even my passion for my former work, the world, and my life ahead of me. Had it all been worth it?

I thought back to our first day of orientation, when one dean, formal yet quirky, a true southern gentleman with a minutely discernible accent that he must have spent some time disguising, stood in front of our ninety-three nervous bodies and reassured us that "over ninety-nine percent of you will graduate." The one who might not finish will have decided that he or she "really doesn't want to practice medicine," he confided. "You have to work to flunk out," he reassured us. And then the next dean, a hybrid East Coast blueblood maverick, repeatedly stressed that if we ever needed academic assistance, it would be provided. "Come to us. Don't wait for us to come to you. Then it's too late," he preemptively admonished. I had been so relieved at that moment, thrilled that I had made the right choice of medical schools. Both deans, who I guessed were from long lines of physicians, were on my side and solidly behind me. Statistics were in my favor, and the deans would help me if necessary.

I returned to the present. I had finally positioned myself by lying sideways over my pile of belongings, carefully adjusting my torso to fit into a valley of clothes. But the lights from the school, which initially had seemed dim, now shone brightly through my windows into my closed eyes. I used books, clothes, and food bags to erect makeshift shades to shield my windows from intruders. But everything kept collapsing. I realized that my barricade might simply draw attention to the contents of my truck. Too tired to care anymore, I covered my head with a blanket. But I was acutely aware that I remained exposed.

Throughout the night, I vacillated between awakened and asleep states, uncertain about each moment. I had flashing thoughts of being robbed, shot, or arrested for sleeping in public. I was startled out of my twisted position five times, once by a large Doberman pinscher that sniffed and then barked at me through my window. Later, three inebriated men woke me as they staggered down the middle of the street, hollering obscenities to the sky. I heard a bottle explode near me. I lay as still as possible as they slowly stumbled by. At other times, my startle reflex fired for no apparent reason.

I finally awoke just before five o'clock, when the early morning light pierced my tenuous barriers, incredulous that I had slept at all. My thoughts of what lay ahead for the day were extinguished by an immediate need to move my truck before I drew suspicion in the neighborhood. As I drove off, I wondered where I would brush my teeth before starting work at the hospital. In my rear view mirror, I could see a puddle trailing off a tree.

· · · · ·

After a series of such nights in my truck, I needed a reprieve. I often fell asleep whenever I sat down, and I found it difficult to remember my patients' names, let alone follow their medical histories or empathize with their complaints. The twenty-four-hour reading room in the undergraduate library seemed to offer a convenient temporary solution. Students had unlimited access, and I had spent at least a week there every exam period, claiming my favorite study table to cram in as much medical knowledge as possible.

I expected to see a familiar face there, a short oval-shaped woman in a thin green windbreaker, with thick brown glasses and silvery hair in a neat bun. Nearly every night, carrying a small canvas briefcase, she would come in between one and two o'clock, as many people were leaving, and disappear into the bathroom for ten minutes before setting up at a desk. She would pull out the same encyclopedic-looking music book from her briefcase, set it in front of her, and, often leaning against the wall, nod off until six or six-thirty, filling the long room with her loud snoring. She curtly told any student who asked that she was studying music. During the day, she would never have drawn attention: she was clean, well-dressed, and intelligent-looking and could easily have been a professor or someone's grandmother or aunt.

It was a quarter to one when I arrived, and I was surprised to find the reading room fairly crowded. As I walked past the rows of unevenly spaced desks toward my study spot, I realized that I was looking for the oval woman. I didn't see her and felt concerned. Though I knew that if I had spotted her that night we might not have spoken to each other, as I never saw her engage with anyone, I still felt some distant connection... as if we would look out for each other through the night... as if we might recognize each other tonight. Maybe she had found a better place to rest her head and find some peace. I hoped so. I contemplated leaving but could not think of any other options. I disappeared into the bathroom for ten minutes with my backpack filled with books and toiletries.

After washing up, I went to my desk, opened a book, and put my forehead down in my folded arms. I was thankful to stretch out my legs. I awoke every hour throughout the night, as if I had set an internal alarm clock, to survey my surroundings. Each time, fewer and fewer people were around. Strangely, when I had taken short study naps here in the past, I seemed to sleep well. But now it was different. A little after six, when I awoke for the last time, two other people were in the room, but still no sign of the oval woman. While I washed up in the bathroom, I wondered if I would ever draw attention as she had done. As I left, I took one final look around, knowing that for some reason this room had changed and I could never return here again.

· · · · ·

I was cramming for a makeup exam that was only four days away, one that I had failed by only one point. I knew that a repeat failure would lead to my dismissal. At some point during that night, I decided to stay in a study room, one of eight small classrooms in the medical school used for lab classes during the day and studying at night. As the night passed, I was interrupted less and less often as students found other available study rooms. When I couldn't read any longer, I considered my options. At first I thought about resting on the tables, but I remembered that they were used for brain dissections and growing microbiological pathogens during the day. The only other option besides the dusty, sticky, stained floors appeared to be the large, black vinyl swivel chairs.

I lined up three in a row but was unable to find a comfortable position. I finally leaned my chair slightly backward in a corner, crossed my outstretched legs, and folded my arms into my chest. I maintained a light nap state until just after two o'clock, when three students entered the room and flipped on the fluorescent overhead lights. My muscles contracted all at once, as if a lightning bolt had hit me. The students were several paces into the room before they saw me, and I could see their incredulous stares. In the same split second that brought them in, they retreated back into the maze of corridors. Though I managed to last two more days there, I finally left the day before the exam and sought another location.

· · · · ·

By now, the days, which once were long on the chaotic wards of the hospital, seemed short in comparison to the nights. I knew I was distracted, so I had my supervisors check my work regularly. Rather than focusing on differential diagnoses of diseases and medical plans for discharging my patients, I often wondered what I would eat that night. My standard lunch and dinner had become peanut butter and jelly bagels with a banana, only $1.08 at the hospital cafeteria, no refrigeration or storage needed. I had to remember which street I had parked my truck on for the day, pay attention to what time I had to move it to avoid getting ticketed, and consider how safe it and my belongings were. I tried to track which of my clothes were in the truck, my hospital locker, or somewhere else. My truck needed to be moved at least twice a day, since parking around the hospital was tightly regulated. But, most important, I wondered whether I would find some rest for the night.

.   .   .   .   .

Besides the nights I spent in my truck, I had the most success finding sleep in call rooms at different hospitals. One medical center where I worked had four rooms for students, two for men and two for women. Each egg-colored room had several sets of tenuously constructed, faux-wood bunk beds that shook like Jell-O. They held multicolored, sagging mattresses stained with who-knew-what. In one room, an entire wall had large holes and chipped paint that revealed about ten shades of green. Each time I inadvertently leaned against the crumbly walls, I wondered how much lead or mold I had inhaled. The holes within the walls revealed an uninsulated center that amplified footsteps and flushing toilet noises from across the building. Each room had a sink and a telephone, the latter a tool to wake the dead and remind us that we were there to work. The archaic heating system transmitted crescendoing bangs during the winter. The rooms were permeated with a distinctive stench, a combination of bleach and blood, seeping from the same linen used throughout the hospital.

Nonetheless, I spent many nights in these rooms, where at least I could wash my hands and lie stretched out in a horizontal position. But they were also used by other students desperate for sleep while on call. A constant flow of people entered and left throughout the night, and the beds shook violently when the seemingly endless pager beeps, buzzes, and rings went off. Many students flipped the lights on and off or propped doors open, flooding the room with sharp light. Others exchanged telephone calls in nonhushed voices throughout the night.

One night, at perhaps three or four in the morning, a student who had been sleeping in the bed next to mine returned from the restroom, came up to my bed, and grabbed my legs. I awoke screaming in a deep visceral tone that I had never heard emerge from my throat. Though he apologized and was snoring away within a short minute—he had probably been sleepwalking or had simply mistaken my bed for his—I was easily startled for the next two days and couldn't return to the call room for some time afterward. That was the closest I had come to suffocating someone with a pillow.

. . . . .

I often found myself wandering along the outskirts of the medical center, near the barren parking lots where one student had recently been robbed at gunpoint, my mind confused about where I was headed, where I might get some rest. One night, I had parked my truck and was getting ready to retire when a vehicle parked behind me turned on its headlights, high-beamed me, and kept them directed at me. I couldn't make out the driver because of the glare, but I could tell from the height of those piercing lights and the dim shadows that my truck was dwarfed by his. I worried that he was driving an old rusted Ford equipped with a gun rack for three rifles. After a full minute, the driver started his truck and slowly pulled up beside me, where he idled for about thirty seconds. I couldn't tell what was happening, but I leaned back, pressing into my seat as far as it would allow. All I heard was the occasional revving of his truck and my shallow, fast breaths. I didn't dare look, as any confrontation might provoke him and lead to a bullet blowing my face open.

He eventually drove off, slowly, deliberately, and as soon as he was out of sight, I took off in the opposite direction to find another place to park. That was the last time I entered that neighborhood.

Another time, I left my truck for two hours, only to return and find my passenger window smashed and half of my belongings stolen. Although I recovered much of my property, which had been stuffed in a dumpster next to a nearby alley, I was unclear why my short white lab coat, surgical reference book, and an old pair of glasses were still missing. I was surprisingly calm as I shook out the broken glass from my truck. But the next day, I was seething with anger when I had to spend an entire day exhuming the thousands of glass shards from my clothes, books, and bench seat before bringing my truck to the repair shop, instead of studying for my repeat surgery exam.

.   .   .   .   .

New acquaintances, patients, or hospital employees occasionally asked me where I lived. I had never realized how personal a question that could be. It struck at my essence, my defined identity up to that point. The truthful answer would open a vista into my life that I was unprepared to expose. I didn't know how to respond. I couldn't name a city, a neighborhood, a street, or an address; I didn't even have a telephone. My only line of communication to the external world had become my pager, an intrusive annoyance that was now my lifeline.

In retrospect, I knew that I had previously asked others to identify their place of residence. "Where do you live?" I once asked a young man, handsome underneath his tattered clothes and layers of mud and dirt. He had just arrived in the emergency room via ambulance after having had a grand mal seizure.

His eyes darted sideways and up, his voice tapered off, and he stuttered, "I live with my mom."

I impatiently repeated, "No, where do you *live?*"

"Can I just go now?" he pleaded.

When I persisted, his face hardened. He glared back at me and gritted out, "What does it matter to you?"

I finally realized that he had no answer. I stopped my intrusive questions and moved on. Later, I discovered that he had just moved from the

Midwest with his mother and younger sister to escape a hopeless future and was now living under a nearby bridge. My sympathy meshed with embarrassment that I had been so insensitive in my haste to evaluate him.

And now I found myself averting my eyes and providing vague responses. But, unlike this young man, I rehearsed an answer until the words flowed effortlessly, as if talking with myself. "I live in San Francisco," I would respond.

"Do you commute ninety minutes each way every day?"

"Mostly," I would say.

"Where do you stay when you don't commute?"

"With friends," I would follow up.

. . . . .

I became familiar with some of the other denizens of the call rooms. One intern lived in a call room until her furniture arrived from the East Coast. She stayed a full month, seemingly unbothered by her circumstances. One student stayed there every third night for months on end; his home was with his wife, who lived five hundred miles away. Another student stayed for three months and even moved her television into a room to try to simulate comfort.

I dreamt one night that the administration found out that I had monopolized the call rooms; the security camera fixed on the hallway had documented my visits and would be used as evidence that I had violated university policy. In my dream, I was charged and dismissed from school for something unrelated to my academic failures: I was dismissed for my character flaws, which allowed me to be living the way I had been.

. . . . .

Eventually, selected parts of my truth came out, and I got varying offers of aid. One classmate offered me his apartment for a month while he was away on an externship, but his roommate, another medical student, felt "uncomfortable" with me staying there. A professor I barely knew offered me a temporary room in her household. And a friend-of-a-friend rented me an extra bedroom in her house for two weeks, but I felt like an intruder. In another person's house, I couldn't relax, cook, or sleep without feeling self-conscious. I felt dependent, reliant. In addition, I knew that my future as a medical student was tenuous at best. I couldn't commit myself to anyone or anything—I needed to be completely free.

. . . . .

One winter morning, I awoke in my truck to a loud, strained, high-pitched noise. My cold-to-touch nose and ears and visible breath reminded me of the outside temperature as I attempted to stop shivering. I was flanked by a damp raincoat, still not dry after the night's storm, a medical dictionary, and mostly empty boxes of crackers, and I was loosely covered by a blanket. I wiped my steamed windshield and spotted the local police flashing their patrol beam across the street. Their lights were directed into the trees, where what seemed like a thousand crows huddled together. The light caused a collective scream from the birds, followed by flurried collisions and a mass exodus into the black sky. What drove the police to do this at 5:30 A.M.? Would they have similarly harassed me if they had seen me? I watched tensely as they continued, helpless to intervene.

After trying to warm up, I decided to head out to the medical school. I biked from my truck, since I hadn't purchased a parking permit at school. I arrived with small amounts of iced breath crusted onto my hair. My hands felt frozen in a clutched position resembling the shape of my handlebars, and my legs felt long, weighted, and stiff. I didn't know if I could manipulate my keys to open the front door, but, to my surprise, it was open, and I waddled in. As I entered the hallways, I felt warmth in the medical school for the first time. It felt good being there, alone, in silence, and I stood there noticing the return of feeling to my fingers and toes.

. . . . .

I'm not sure whether I'm dozing or waking, or how much time has passed, but I've been covered by a quilt that holds my warm body just right. My back is now perfectly contoured with the sofa, and I'm lulled into full consciousness by the aroma of a cup of hot cocoa set beside me.

I sit silent and still. My eyes fix on the pink tree, and I imagine the spirits sitting next to the bright flowers, holding their fists tight, signaling me to keep going. I turn and gaze at Jeanine, and then, without warning, several tears drop from my eyes and I'm confused. I haven't had the luxury to reflect on the past seven years, the time it took me to complete the prerequisite basic science courses and medical school classes. I think about the time I've lost, and whether I might have comforted Chopper during his thirty-second year, his last, before he died of AIDS, or might have noticed Mary becoming withdrawn before she attempted suicide. I think about the weekend dinner parties I had missed, lounging at Lana's house on Sundays, walking the beach with Nancy. I wonder whether I will ever have time again with my family and friends. I think about the years during which I could have continued research, political lobbying, and volunteer work. I think about the years in which I could have started a family, gardened, built a home and a life for myself. But instead, I had used up everything while struggling to survive in an environment and life that I now despise.

And what did I gain? The "privilege" of working thirty-six hour shifts, and sometimes one-hundred-hour weeks, and becoming so tired that I would fall asleep standing and almost while driving, endangering my life and the lives of innocent bystanders. The "gift" of giving up all my personal time, at the expense of my family and friends, to be among strangers. The "honor" of entering a profession where public humiliation is the mode of educational training. The ability to "help" patients, the same ones to whom I cannot devote my full attention because I am so overwhelmed, overworked, and frustrated. All of this while paying more than one hundred thousand dollars for an education with no guarantee of even graduating and an uncertain future career in a crumbling national health care system. I mourn my lost life, want enough time to remember the reasons why I entered medicine. I want to see a future.

· · · · ·

During my last two days with Jeanine, we sprawl out on her sofa, where sometimes her enormous Maine Coon cat warms my lap and legs. We talk for hours, laugh, and eat hot home-cooked meals. And I sleep— long, hard, and deep—as I used to, before medical school.

· · · · ·

It's summer now, eight months since I moved into my truck. And I've still got another year of school left. My belongings remain in storage boxes in different locations throughout San Francisco. I'm writing this on a train going from Washington, D.C., to New York. I have no reason for this visit, other than curiosity. It has been thirteen years since I last lived in New York and seven since I last visited. I wonder whether the city will look different, whether I will remember the neighborhoods. I've lost contact with everyone I once knew there. As I look out through the train window at the miles of abandoned brick houses zipping by, burned and boarded up, aligned in perfect rows on what were once perfect streets, I wonder whether I will ever return to medical school.

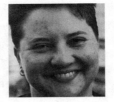

SOMETIMES, ALL YOU CAN DO IS LAUGH

M edical school makes it so damn hard to keep your sense of humor. Ironically, it gives you so much new comedic material at the same time. I mean, when you think about it, having to memorize the names of all the complement fragments (you know, those funny little chemicals) is pretty funny. It's almost as if someone designed them to be ridiculous: C4b2a? C3bBb? C3PO? R2D2? RU-SR-E-S? Who are they kidding? I half expect to see Allen Funt popping out of a bush screaming, "Smile, you're on *Candid Camera!*"

And memorizing the genome of the adenovirus? I don't *want* to know the genome of the adenovirus. I'm glad somebody knows it. And it's fine with me if they use my tax dollars to research it, but I don't need to commit it to memory. I might forget my phone number.

I have a theory, which someday I am going to publish for my Ph.D., that there are only five enzymes. Each time they find one of them in some novel location or reaction, they name it something else. And they know it, too; it's all an elaborate plot to generate material for Ph.D. dissertations. But what about the poor medical students who have to learn them all? Does anyone care about *us?* Hell, no. If we refuse to memorize the enzymes, there are hundreds of other students desperate enough to get into medical school who would gladly memorize them. They're just a FAFSA—a Free Application for Federal Student Aid—away from filling your spot, anyway.

After fifteen months, I believe that I have discovered the purpose of medical school (that is, if *Candid Camera* isn't behind it). The system of medical education is a scheme funded by an insurance consortium to desensitize trainees to inanity, repetition, fatigue, and bureaucracy. It was designed so that when we're out in the real world, we'll be too incapacitated to ask the right questions. Questions like, why will insurers sometimes pay for inpatient artificial respiration for someone in a persistent vegetative state but not for hospice care? Why do insurers pay for Viagra more often than for birth control pills? Why do physicians have to get approval from insurance company–hired clerks and nurses to order a simple study like a CAT scan? (I always thought it was the doctors who were supposed to know which tests were medically appropriate. Do these clerks and nurses have degrees higher than a physician's?) And why do insurance companies spend millions to help elect politicians, who then give them kickbacks? For that matter, why did we spend forty million dollars for Kenneth Starr to investigate the White House sex scandal when we don't have the budget to provide preventative medical care to children?

What was I saying? Oh, yes, medical school. It is a *true* test of my hippocampal function. But the real craziness is being immersed in the dominant culture day after day. While I realize that there aren't exactly a lot of thirty-year-old lesbian mothers attending medical school in Ohio, it would be nice not to be the only one. Maybe then I wouldn't have to explain artificial insemination to someone with a degree in biology. Maybe then I wouldn't have to announce over and over again that even though I don't have a husband, I have a perfectly legitimate family who needs me. Maybe then I could get my financial aid budget adjusted to reflect the fact that I have two kids. (Plastic dinosaurs can get expensive, you know.)

And maybe then my sexual orientation and role as a parent wouldn't creep into my daily decisions. Should I skip the transplant immunology lecture to go to parents' night at preschool? Are they (the kids, not the immunologists) being psychologically damaged by my absence? Is this a good time in my career to e-mail the dean to complain about the hideous lack of gay and lesbian visibility in the curriculum? (Yes, folks, there are lesbian and gay people in Ohio, and one of them might be your doctor! Or your patient!) Should I be outraged at the closeted members of my class (not to mention closeted faculty, interns, and residents) because I have to stand alone as the only "out" person? And, most important, do I have to shave my legs for physical diagnosis lab?

Every Tuesday afternoon in physical diagnosis lab, we would break up into small gender-segregated groups, change into hospital gowns, and pretend to examine each other. I did decide to shave my legs so that I wouldn't freak out any of my straight classmates, but I couldn't bring myself to do the same to my armpits. So, week after week, I sat in my hospital gown on the table in the pathology lab room with my arms firmly at my sides. I'd think about how I really should work out more and how I needed a method to avoid staring at anyone's breasts while still remembering the lung exam. I would spend the whole time worrying that everyone else was worrying about getting undressed in front of me. I was angry that any of that even mattered. Like straight people don't ever look at other same-sex naked people! Still, I would get dressed behind the door in the bathroom.

Once, while demonstrating proper chest auscultation technique, our instructor completely removed the gown worn by one of my classmates. The poor woman just sat there shivering, while we gathered around and tried to look attentive without acknowledging the bare facts in front of us. It's hard to believe that our instructor kept talking on and on about lung sounds, as if we were all listening. Instead, we were all thanking God the whole time that it wasn't us sitting there shivering.

And then there's the strange but incontrovertible fact that I seem to be the only one disturbed by the gender and sexuality issues in the curriculum. Consider, for example, an infectious disease "specialist" who ascribes the transmission of some intestinal parasites exclusively to gay men via a certain sexual activity—as if heterosexuals don't know the pleasures of anal sex. (And what about the "straight" ones who are engaging in homosexual sex?) Do you think it would be acceptable for medical students to comment, "Ew-w-w," "Aw-w-w," or "Yuck," if they were instead talking about missionary intercourse? And no one ever points out that heterosexual vaginal intercourse spreads much more disease (including HIV). When was the last time you saw a lesbian with complications from an unintended, unwanted, or ectopic pregnancy?

Or how about the first-year anatomy text wherein the author reassuringly goes to great lengths (!) to point out (!) that individual differences in flaccid penis size are more than corrected for during erection. In other words, if it's not as big as the one you notice on the guy next to you in the shower (or while changing for physical diagnosis lab), you don't have to worry, because it'll grow all the more when the time comes. Predictably, the corresponding commentary in the female perineum section explains condescendingly that in fact there exist virgins without intact hymens. In other words, a perforated hymen need not be taken as proof of sexual activity—as if proper women are concerned only about the appearance of virginity and not with pleasure or function. Pointing all this out to several of my classmates resulted in blank stares. It's exhausting. Sometimes, all you can do is laugh.

I haven't felt this out of place since high school. I couldn't keep my mouth shut then, either. Last week, I had the nerve to suggest over stale donuts in my problem-based learning session on neonatology that maybe it isn't such a good idea to go around cutting off the foreskins of perfectly healthy baby boys who aren't able to consent to elective surgery. From the looks on everyone's faces, you'd think no one in medical school had ever said "foreskin" at breakfast before, much less suggested campaigning against a billable service. I wonder what will happen when that topic is broached again—say, by the first Monday morning patient? Or is it just that every male in Ohio is happily circumcised?

I seem to have joined some kind of private club: an Orwellian sort of village, where we do things simply because we've always done them that way. I guess that would be okay if it was working, but what if it's not? What if the heretics are right?

Take a look into our medical past. One pre-antibiotic treatment for syphilis was to induce fever by inoculating the patient with *Plasmodium falciparum* (malaria), let the fever rise to the point of delirium, and then administer quinine (poison, an antidote for malaria) to get rid of the parasite. (This actually worked, to some extent, and won Viennese psychiatrist Wagner von Jauregg the Nobel Prize in 1927.) This "treatment" method was a vast improvement over the previously popular treatment for syphilis, which was to fumigate the patient with poisonous mercury vapor until his teeth fell out. This had the added benefit of rendering the poor guy so disabled that he'd promise never to have sex again if only the doctors would stay away from him. (I'm using the masculine pronoun here because in many cases they didn't waste the cinnabar, the raw material from which mercury was extracted, on syphilitic women, unless there was some reason to believe that a particular woman had been innocently infected—like from a toilet seat, I guess.)

Here's some further perspective on our scientific "advances." It took more than four hundred years from the first recorded case of syphilis until the discovery of the causative agent *Treponema pallidum*. Another twenty-three years passed before Alexander Fleming discovered penicillin in his petri dish (though he didn't get the Nobel until 1945); and forty-four more years went by before the end of the Tuskegee Syphilis Study, in which black men with syphilis were diagnosed but not treated, in order to "study" the long-term effects of syphilis.[1] (And some people wonder why

1. The U.S. Public Health Service conducted the Tuskegee Syphilis Study in Alabama, from 1932 to 1972. The six hundred subjects, of whom about four hundred had syphilis, were all African American men, most of them poor. They were told only that they were suffering from "bad blood" and were not informed of the study's actual purpose. By design, they were never given the penicillin that could have cured their illness. See A. M. Brandt, "Racism and Research: The Case of the Tuskegee Syphilis Study," *Hastings Center Report* 8, no. 6 (1978): 21–29; J. H. Jones, *Bad Blood: The Tuskegee Syphilis Experiment* (New York: Free Press, 1993); and S. M. Reverby, ed., *Tuskegee Truths: Rethinking the Tuskegee Syphilis Study* (Chapel Hill: University of North Carolina Press, 2000).

African Americans don't trust the medical profession.) Yet last year there were 4,013 cases of syphilis in the United States, despite the fact that it is virtually 100 percent curable by a single dose of penicillin.

Given the paradigm of medical science, the structure and content of medical school curriculum, and the misinformation on gender and sexual issues, I'll bet the heretics *are* right. Maybe what we really need now is a bunch of uppity queer science geeks to get this thing back on course (go ACT UP!). Just wait 'till they see who I'm gonna pick to mentor.

Now that I've somehow become a part of this private club, I'll let you in on a big secret: medical school is *not* intellectually difficult. Everyone says it is, because it's a big pain in the ass, and they want you to feel sorry for them. But you don't have to be a genius, and you don't have to have any special skills. Hell, you don't even have to be good with people. You just have to mindlessly memorize minutiae, know whose butt to kiss, refrain from asking any questions, and collect all the right signatures. In the process, though, you might learn something about the profession (and maybe even a little pathology, if you're paying attention to the professors).

Maybe I shouldn't complain. After all, medical education has given me a lot to think about. For instance, why are so many pathological findings named after food? Nutmeg liver? Cheesy granuloma? Red currant jelly sputum? Is this a way of forcing us all into dieting? And if hospitals are so full of antibiotic-resistant germs, why do we send everyone without an intact immune system to one? And whose idea was this fee-for-service thing, anyway?

Just the other day, one of my colleagues, fresh from Economics 101, was patiently explaining how we should just charge cash for health services and that eventually the free market will drive the prices down. I pointed out that that's what got us here in the first place and that, except for electronics, the price of everything only goes up, not down. And anyway, Ronald Reagan isn't president anymore, so we needn't be toeing that old line. Then I moved in for the kill. If we orchestrate a drop in health care fees to a level where everyone can afford them—until an office visit is, say, the price of an oil change—how will we pay the insurance company presidents their thirty-million-dollar-a-year salaries, build that brand-new hospital building named after some old rich guy, *and* have enough to support the thousands of lawyers who make their living by suing doctors for malpractice? When I'm old enough to run for president (2004), my campaign platform will be based on three simple policy changes: outlaw handguns, legalize marijuana, and use the money we save to create National Health Care.

All in all, maybe medical school isn't so bad. I have met some interesting people; there are lots of fun, gruesome slides of tropical parasitic infections; and, if you memorize the weekly medicine grand rounds schedule, you can get a free sandwich and maybe even a drug company highlighter. And, let's see, you can walk around in the short white coat feeling self-important—at least in comparison to the pre-meds. Oh, and there is the ever-present "carrot" dangled before you hinting that someday, if you manage to tread water long enough, you might be able to do something useful, or at least comforting, for your patients. Most days, I'm just too tired to wonder whether this is true, so I keep dragging myself to the library in the hope that one day I'll look up and be standing at graduation. Or, better yet, talking to a patient who is healthier because she tripped over the phone book and landed on my name. Sometimes, all you can do is laugh.

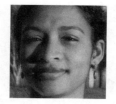

A PRAYER FROM A CLOSETED CHRISTIAN

Dear Lord,

Please forgive me, for I have failed You. I look back on my three-plus years of medical school, and I am ashamed. You gave Your life for me on the cross, and I have only now begun to stand up for You.

I began medical school with every intention of staying close to You, no matter what. But it became harder as I struggled to keep up with all the material I had to learn. I fear that, in my worry, I put You second. I chose studying over church on Sunday. I could have made it to evening services, but then I needed to study more. The Christian Medical and Dental Society was a great opportunity for me, but somehow I never got to more than one meeting. I always seemed to have slides to review or cases to read. Or else I ran out for a quick lunch and just forgot about the meeting.

Thank You for embracing me during my second year when I sought solace in Your arms. I was angry with school, angry that it kept me away from my grandmother's funeral in the Caribbean. I could have gone and then taken makeup exams later, but I couldn't handle the stress of school and a family tragedy all at once. All of my anger descended on medical school; I thought that it kept me from being with her, comforting her as she left this earth, standing and holding my mother's hand as she wept at the grave site. I ran back to You because I couldn't stand to be at school. I needed You. Church once again became a priority, and although I studied harder than ever, I made time for You. And I did well, better than I had during the first year.

My third year brought new challenges to my faith in You. Church wasn't always possible because I worked on Sundays. As my church family sang praises to You, I presented cases on rounds, hoping that my delivery was slowly coming to resemble a good presentation. Sometimes I made it back in time for evening services, but most times I returned home to collapse into bed. I tried to read Your word every night, but I was on call sometimes every fourth night and forgot to take my Bible with me to the hospital. Other times I remembered You as my eyes slowly shut, sleep tempting me as I tried to read up on patients for the next day. As I dozed off, I caught glimpses of my Bible from the corners of half-shut eyes. I told myself I would read in the morning, but my Bible always sat unopened as I raced out the door into the blackness of morning on my way to "pre-round" on my patients (that is, to collect their vital signs, do a physical exam, and summarize the events of the past twenty-four hours before the medical team met to discuss the daily plan for each patient).

My true test of faith lay in working with the senior members of my team. I didn't ask for all Sundays off when given the chance, afraid that I would be told it was unfair to the other students. You know I believe in prayer. I believe that it can change everything. But when the senior resident made fun of a patient's religious beliefs, I did not defend You.

"What? Are we going to start praying at every person's bedside now?" he asked rhetorically, but I remained silent.

I wanted to share Your word as You commanded Your disciples, but somehow it didn't seem appropriate, as if I had to obey an unspoken law about separation of church and medicine. I knew Your law was more important, but I was afraid. Would the team reprimand me if I mentioned Christianity? Or laugh? What if my patients brought it up first?

I remained unsure on the inside, uncommitted on the outside. And I was ashamed. I had become a closeted Christian.

But then, Lord, do You remember Mr. Elijah? He was that southern Santa Claus–looking man with colon cancer. He helped me find the courage to acknowledge You, fully and publicly. During rounds one day, Mr. Elijah told me, "Me and my friends used to go swimmin' in North Carolina where I grew up. We'd spend all day there divin' and playin'..." He laughed and added, "sometimes with no clothes on." Suddenly he stopped and looked at me with his eyes welling up. "You know, I would do anything to dip my toes in that sweet Carolina water again."

I didn't know what to say.

He started crying but shook his head in determination. "But I believe I can beat this, because God can heal me, and with Him anything and everything is possible."

I wanted desperately to hold his hand and reply, "Yes, anything is possible with God. I believe in miracles too." I wanted to offer to pray with him right there. But I knew that the team of doctors was standing right behind me, so I said nothing. I left the room weighted down with disappointment. I was a Christian—why didn't I pray with him? This good man shared Your love with me, and I didn't return it.

I was crying inside, Lord, and that night I cried with my Bible in my hands. This was not what I was supposed to have become. I had allowed my work as a medical student and my fears as a junior team member to interfere with my Christian life. I had failed to share Your word. I had neglected to keep Your last commandment: *Go ye therefore and teach all nations . . .*

That was two weeks ago, Lord. Mr. Elijah came back today. He told me that he was still hanging on and that he had been forced to cancel a camping trip to North Carolina to come here. But he'd make it there the next time. "All with God's help," he said. "He can do anything."

I squeezed his shoulder, and this time I responded: "Yes, He can." And, Lord, then I offered to pray for him and told him to keep his faith up. When I left his room, I felt renewed. Mr. Elijah reminded me to walk Your path no matter what others think.

So, Lord, tonight I'm praying for Mr. Elijah, that You will make him well or welcome him into Your kingdom, according to Your will. From now on, Lord, I will affirm that with You all things are possible. I will offer Your hope to my patients and never remain silent when I ought to witness to Your truth. Help me to stand firm in my faith and never to deny You. I pray this in Jesus' name. Amen.

. . . . .

I am now a fourth-year student and will soon be a physician. After my experience with Mr. Elijah, I began to use phrases that would be encouraging to all my patients but that I hoped would be recognizable as Christian to other Christians. With them, I pray, and I remind them to believe in the miracle of God's love. I give my patients their medical prognosis as I've been taught to, but I always add the words, " . . . but we cannot tell for sure what will happen" to remind them and myself that, next to the power of God, medical science is weak indeed.

Also, I feel more at peace combining my work as a physician with my Christian faith. Sometimes people ask, "How can you be a Christian *and* a scientist? Don't you know that medical theories are based on evolution?" Another common question is, "Isn't it a little hypocritical to say that God heals people when you are going into medicine for the same reason?"

I do not believe in evolution. I believe in a God who created earth and everything on it. I believe in an afterlife. I believe that as a physician, I will serve as God's instrument, and *through* my work *He* will heal people. I am a Christian. I don't play God; I work for Him. I am at a point where I can speak to senior team members who argue with a Jehovah's Witness patient refusing a blood transfusion but make no attempt to address her beliefs. And I can openly disagree with the resident who remarks that "religion is the opiate of the masses." Every day, patients freely share their faith with me, and I am amazed at the depth of their faith in love and in God.

. . . . .

Dear Lord, devout is what I want to be for You, at work and elsewhere, any time, any place. Thank You for having patience and for giving me the strength to make You proud. Amen.

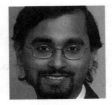

SEEING WITH NEW EYES

HOW AYURVEDA TRANSFORMED MY LIFE

I n June 1999, after a year of medical school at the University of California at San Francisco, I began my study of Ayurveda, the traditional medical system of India. Ayurveda, which derives its name from a Sanskrit phrase meaning "knowledge of life," is the oldest known system of medicine. Its principles were first recorded in the Vedas, the original Hindu scriptures, more than five thousand years ago.

While I strongly believe in Western allopathic medicine, I am also aware of its limitations and feel that it may not meet the needs of all patients. For several years, I had been intrigued by alternative medicine, especially Ayurveda. As books and workshops piqued my interest, I began to sense that it had much to offer in areas that were not addressed by allopathic medicine.

Although I was raised in a traditional Indian family, I did not have any significant exposure to Ayurveda while growing up. My interest in alternative approaches to healing developed during college, when I began exploring ultimate questions of life and reality and started to read about Indian philosophy and spirituality. I was especially intrigued by Yoga, a set of diverse practices designed to integrate physical, mental, and spiritual health. Through Yoga, I became interested in Ayurveda and tried to evaluate the effects of these practices on myself. I became vegetarian, began practicing meditation daily, and made other Ayurvedic diet and lifestyle changes that completely and irrevocably transformed my life. I felt a sense of balance, peace, and vitality that I had never imagined possible. After experiencing firsthand the power of Ayurveda and Yoga, I knew that I wanted to somehow incorporate these systems into my future practice of medicine.

Between my first and second years of medical school, I found a center that taught classical Ayurveda, while adapting it to modern times: the Arya Vaidya Chikitsalayam (Ayurvedic hospital) and Research Institute, located in Coimbatore, South India. I registered for a six-week summer introductory course in Ayurveda and Yoga.

. . . . .

I arrived in Coimbatore at the end of June and met my classmates, one American and six British students. On our first day, we were presented with an ambitious weekly schedule, featuring thirty-three hours of instruction that included seminars and interactive workshops, daily Yoga practice, and lessons in Sanskrit. I found the teachers exceptional, my classmates congenial, and the material fascinating.

We began by studying Ayurvedic anatomy and physiology. Then, in the second week, we participated in interactive workshops that allowed us both to provide and to experience Ayurvedic therapies. Once I volunteered to receive a type of bodywork known as Pirichil-Dhara. In this treatment, warm medicated oil was continuously poured over and massaged into my entire body by four therapists, each responsible for one quadrant of my body. Meanwhile, another attendant gently rocked a clay pot suspended overhead, pouring oil in a mesmerizing rhythm across my forehead. The hour-long session was unforgettable and deeply healing.

Other classes introduced us to herbal pharmacology, pathology, and diet and lifestyle recommendations. We also took some field trips that helped us appreciate the context in which Ayurveda is practiced. We toured an Ayurvedic pharmaceutical company and visited two herbal gardens to study plants used in treatment.

One day near the end of the summer, an instructor was conducting a review session. As I sat with the other students, I suddenly had a revelation about Ayurveda. I realized its all-encompassing nature. It integrates all aspects of life: physical, emotional, and spiritual daily rhythms and life cycles, other animals and plants, seasonal changes, and even the very energy of Life itself, known as Prana. I saw how everything fit together in remarkable concinnity and completeness. I ceased listening to the teacher; time seemed to stop. I felt as if I had fallen in love. I knew then that this summer course was only the beginning of a lifetime relationship with Ayurveda.

Later, when I described this incident to the medical director of the institute, he replied that he had had a similar experience in Ayurvedic medical school. He told me that the completeness and perfection of Ayurvedic theory are often attributed to its divine origin. Ancient sages in India formulated its principles through deep meditation and intuition, invoking Brahma, the Hindu god of creation. The director said that many Ayurvedic doctors experience moments of insight into its beauty during their training, inspiring them to commit their lives to Ayurveda. I wondered whether I had had a similar experience.

In any case, I began to appreciate Ayurveda as much more than a system of medicine. It is a combination of science, religion, and philosophy that may best be described as a way of life. It offers a comprehensive, practical science for bringing the individual into complete balance on multiple levels. I was learning how to heal disease, but, more important, I was learning how to live in balance.

. . . . .

When I returned from India, I began to perceive Western medicine in a new way. Because I had been immersed in a different system, I was able to critically analyze allopathic medicine with more objectivity and detachment. It seemed easier to step back and view things as an outsider. I felt as though I had a secret advantage, in the form of a new way of looking at things, a completely different perspective that I could draw on when necessary. This gave me a sense of freedom and self-confidence and made me less concerned that important parts of myself would change during the "conditioning" process of medical training.

I began to analyze allopathic training. The traditional Indian approach to Ayurvedic education differs fundamentally from Western medical education. It emphasizes the teaching of moral and spiritual wisdom in addition to professional knowledge. Skills for living are introduced, along with facts and concepts. The instructors at the institute had sometimes taught by relating stories or personal experiences. The teacher-student relationship is crucial, and students are given the flexibility to guide the class content through questions and comments. This approach originates in the guru-disciple tradition of teaching in India, a philosophy dramatically different from the one I was accustomed to in my U.S. medical school.

The Ayurvedic approach to science is also different, though no less rigorous than the allopathic paradigm. I found Ayurvedic theory logical enough to satisfy my Western training. Observation and analysis are modes of inquiry common to both traditions, except that the means sometimes vary. For example, Ayurvedic reasoning often proceeds from macrocosm to microcosm, relying on an intuitive understanding of the whole to define the parts. Conversely, Western science usually begins with smaller units and progresses to larger structures, believing that understanding all the parts leads to understanding the whole. This difference reflects the holistic basis of Ayurvedic thinking and, in contrast, the more mechanistic and reductionist Western approach.

Hence, I began to reconsider the concept of specialization within allopathic training. After my summer in India, I felt that specializing would not be consistent with my new view of the body. Ayurveda emphasizes the interconnectedness of the human being. It states that a disease may manifest itself outwardly at one point in the body but originate in a completely different, seemingly unrelated part. One must therefore treat the whole person in order to treat the disease successfully. I knew intellectually that this view need not be inconsistent with specialty training, but nonetheless I realized that primary care, with its generalist approach, would be my path.

Another aspect of allopathic medicine that I reexamined was its pharmacology. At the beginning of my second year of medical school, when I first picked up our pharmacology syllabus, I was struck by the cover illustration. It depicted a mock battle scene, complete with trenches, forts, and barbed wire, in which bacteria were engaged in combat with soldiers representing various antibiotics. As the semester progressed, I noticed that the language of war and violence was pervasive. Phrases like "assaulted by invading antigens" and "war between man and microbe" were not unusual. Words such as "attack," "combat," "target," and even "armamentarium" were common. I realized that this was the standard working vocabulary of pharmacology.

I became increasingly uncomfortable with the implications of this type of language. The military model is inconsistent with the way I now view health and illness. I conceive of perfect health as the natural state of the individual. I believe that medicines that support and strengthen the body's self-healing abilities are often effective, with minimal adverse effects. To me, the language of violence, associated with negative feelings such as aggression and fear, is not in line with my highest ideals of healing. It does not seem to foster a healthy way of understanding medicine. I dislike the fact that the war metaphor is used to describe the fundamental basis of allopathic medicine.

.   .   .   .   .

During my summer in India, an Ayurveda teacher told a story about a village that had problems with mosquitoes. The villagers developed a chemical spray to kill the insects. They sprayed whenever they saw them, and the mosquitoes disappeared. It appeared that the problem had been solved. However, a few weeks later, the mosquitoes began to reappear, and the villagers were puzzled. Finally, someone discovered a pond of stagnant water near the village that was the breeding ground for all the mosquitoes. When this pond was drained, they found a permanent solution to the mosquito problem.

My teacher explained that the chemical sprays were analogous to Western antibiotics. Ayurveda believes that a more effective strategy is to address the root cause, represented by the pond in the story, that creates a predisposition to the problem. Ayurveda states that a person who is in good health, and living in balance on all levels, will not usually fall sick, even with exposure to most infectious pathogens. Thus, the Ayurvedic pharmacopoeia does not have equivalents to Western antibiotics. Ayurvedic treatment does not fight organisms that cause infection. Antibiotics are seen as a treatment of an already manifesting illness, and thus they may be of only temporary benefit. Instead, Ayurvedic treatment seeks to strengthen the body's own restorative powers and to correct the underlying imbalance that allowed the individual to become ill in the first place.

I am not suggesting that antibiotics are unnecessary. I believe that they are important, have saved many lives, and have their place in the treatment of certain infections. But my hope is that other approaches, such as Ayurveda, can help us strengthen our immune systems and live healthy, balanced lives so that we can decrease the incidence of infectious disease, thereby reducing antibiotic usage.

. . . . .

Sometimes I share these ideas with my classmates in allopathic medicine. Their reactions are mixed, but often my views are seen as quite foreign and unusual. However, discussions with classmates help me to see things from a fresh perspective and to appreciate positive characteristics of allopathic medicine that I sometimes overlook. They help me to moderate and balance my views when I become overly focused on alternative medicine.

Occasionally, someone becomes defensive and feels the need to stand up for allopathic medicine, although I emphasize that my goal is never to attack it, but to examine it critically and think about areas for potential improvement. A few of my classmates are passionate scientists and believe that science should be used to examine all phenomena. With them, I agree that scientific research is essential, but I also try to point out the limitations of science and explain that it is only one tool we can use to understand the world. I often find it difficult to bridge the gap between these different perspectives, however.

Fortunately, there are several students with whom I share many values and beliefs. One of them spent some time researching Ayurveda in India before beginning medical school. Another, who is very interested in homeopathy, successfully raised a child without the use of a single antibiotic. With these classmates, I openly share my views on integrative medicine, a holistic, relationship-centered approach to medicine that synthesizes the best of alternative and conventional modalities.

One of the reasons I chose to attend the University of California at San Francisco was its relative openness to alternative and integrative medicine. As a part of the standard curriculum, five elective alternative medicine courses are offered, and the new Osher Center for Integrative Medicine was recently established. During my first year, I became involved with a student organization known as the Integrative Medicine Network at UCSF.

I worked with a group of students to organize the first UCSF Integrative Medicine Forum, a two-day multidisciplinary conference. Our goals were to raise awareness about integrative medicine and the key issues in the field and to elucidate the practice of alternative therapies through interactive workshops. In planning the curriculum, we were mindful that it would be the first such conference at our campus. When selecting the topics for small group workshops, we chose modalities that were relatively well established and widely known, such as acupuncture, chiropractic medicine, and Yoga. We decided not to include therapies that were considered more esoteric and might alienate the more skeptical attendees—for example, energy healing techniques such as Reiki or Therapeutic Touch. We also knew that we had to speak the language with which most attendees would be comfortable—the language of science and research. Therefore, we tried to select presenters who had experience speaking to physicians and could explain their work in a scientific way. In addition, we scheduled a panel discussion about exploring challenges in investigating the efficacy of alternative therapies using conventional methodology.

After months of planning, the forum was a great success. The event featured forty-four speakers and drew nearly two hundred fifty attendees, including students from other medical schools. Several faculty members volunteered to speak, and a number of campus funding sources contributed. Many students, staff, and faculty attended, and feedback about the conference was mostly positive. Overall, it set a good precedent and was followed by forums in 2000 and 2001 that each attracted more than four hundred attendees.

In addition, I took one year off between my second and third years of medical school to work as the education coordinator at the Osher Center for Integrative Medicine. By organizing professional conferences, workshops, and classes for students and community members, I was able to help increase awareness about alternative medicine in a meaningful and fulfilling way. I worked with several outstanding physician mentors who gave me invaluable guidance and encouraged me to continue following my heart as I pursued training in other systems of healing.

I sometimes forget that many at my medical school are skeptical of integrative medicine, because I am often around people who share my interests. I forget that we are not representative of the whole medical school community. For example, during one anatomy class, the professor discussed the treatment of pain. He spoke highly of the allopathic treatments. He then proceeded to list a number of alternative treatments for pain and dismissed each one, attributing any demonstrated effect to a placebo response. He singled out acupuncture and made two incorrect assertions that supposedly proved that the effectiveness of acupuncture was based on the placebo effect. And though he listened to contrary viewpoints after class, he did not seem convinced. Overall, however, I am very grateful that my medical school offers more resources and fosters more interest in integrative medicine than many other schools.

. . . . .

Eventually, I want to integrate the clinical practices of Ayurveda and allopathic medicine. I believe that each represents a different but equally valid way of understanding health and that both have a great deal to contribute to the future of health care. I find it striking how illnesses that are not easily treated in one system are often extremely responsive to treatment in the other tradition. Thus, the two approaches can represent a remarkably powerful combination. I believe it is possible to bring together the best elements of both medical systems in a synergistic manner. This synthesis may also help me to harmonize the two divergent but equally important aspects of my Indian American identity.

One of the most valuable ideas I gained from my study of Ayurveda is the emphasis on self-transformation and healing the healer. Ayurveda features a strong focus on personal and spiritual growth, living a life of balance, and sincerely working to heal oneself first during the process of training. This emphasis has transformed my experience within medical school. While I still concentrate on learning all the medical facts and knowledge, I also place a great deal of attention on my own physical and emotional health. I try to continue growing as a person in other ways and seek to develop my compassion and spirituality. I feel that these perspectives will enable me to sustain a long and productive career in medicine and will help prevent the burnout that is becoming increasingly common among physicians.

The Charaka Samhita, a classical Ayurvedic text compiled in 1500 B.C. and still used today, states, "There is no end to the learning of Ayurveda." The same could be said of allopathic medicine. I believe that the path of becoming an integrative healer will be a lifelong process of learning, personal growth, and transformation. I look forward to it.

PART THREE: CONFRONTED

A t the beginning of the nineteenth century, medicine in the United States encompassed the practices of Native American doctors, homeopaths, botanists, bonesetters, abortionists, cancer doctors, midwives, and others.[1] Women served as lay practitioners and had provided most home medical care since colonial times. Over the ensuing decades, however, and into the twentieth century, medicine evolved into a homogeneous, highly regulated, professionalized, and elite entity. Medical schools developed stricter entrance requirements, a greater emphasis on expensive scientific laboratories, and affiliations with wealthy universities; and they charged higher tuition. From the middle of the nineteenth century until the early 1960s, women constituted no more than 6 percent of all medical students, except during World War II, when doctors were badly needed.[2] With the exception of historically black institutions—most notably, Howard University College of Medicine and Meharry Medical College, the longest surviving

1. P. Starr, *The Social Transformation of American Medicine* (New York: Basic Books, 1982), 47–50, describes a variety of these medical practices.

2. For information about the numbers of women in medicine, see M. R. Walsh, *"Doctors Wanted, No Women Need Apply": Sexual Barriers in the Medical

such schools—medical schools did not welcome African Americans.[3] No financial aid system existed. Accordingly, medical schools educated primarily the privileged: mostly white men of higher social classes who could afford to pay the expensive tuition.[4]

The social and political upheaval of the 1960s finally forced medical schools to begin admitting a more diverse body of students. The Civil Rights Act of 1964 prohibited federally funded programs, including many medical schools, from discriminating on the basis of race, but it took another decade to significantly affect medical school demographics. In 1968, minority medical students (African American, Chicano, Native American, and mainland Puerto Rican) accounted for only 3 percent of all new entering medical students, or 292 people.[5] In 1972, as a result of the feminist movement of the 1960s and 1970s, Congress passed Title IX, barring sexual discrimination in admissions and

---

Profession, 1835–1975 (New Haven: Yale University Press, 1977), 178–269. Also see D. G. Johnson, *U.S. Medical Students, 1950–2000: A Companion Fact Book for Physicians in the Making* (Washington, D.C.: Association of American Medical Colleges, 1983), 66–67.

3. The barriers faced by African American medical school applicants are discussed in K. M. Ludmerer, *Time to Heal: American Medical Education from the Turn of the Century to the Era of Managed Care* (New York: Oxford University Press, 1999), 63.

4. Concerning the factors contributing to the traditional makeup of medical school classes, see Ludmerer, *Time to Heal*, 63–65; V. W. Lippard, *A Half-Century of American Medical Education: 1920–1970* (New York: Josiah Macy Jr. Foundation, 1974), 32; and Starr, *Social Transformation of American Medicine*, 124.

5. These statistics are drawn from L. Robinson, ed., *AAMC Data Book: Statistical Information Related to Medical Students and Teaching Hospitals* (Washington, D.C.: Association of American Medical Colleges, 2001), 12–13. Note that the discussion here refers to groups that would become "underrepresented minorities," a term that does not include Asians. The history of Asians in medical education is unique because, although they are considered "minorities" in the larger American culture and are treated as such, their numbers have been overrepresented in medical schools, relative to their numbers in the population, for several decades.

employment in any institution of higher education that received federal funds. Women began to enter medicine in record numbers. By 1975, women, mostly white, accounted for 20 percent of new medical school admits, and minorities had increased to 9 percent.[6]

Doors also began to open for other traditionally excluded or stigmatized groups. In 1974, after pressure from the gay and lesbian community, the American Psychiatric Association finally removed homosexuality as a defined psychiatric illness. Since sexual orientation has never been recorded as a statistic in medical school admissions, the impact of this change is unknown. But it is likely to have been reflected in greater tolerance or encouragement for lesbian, gay, and bisexual individuals as prospective medical students. More recently, the passage of the Americans with Disabilities Act in 1992 forced schools to make reasonable accommodations for applicants and students with mental or physical disabilities.

National and local lobbying, the passage of historic legislation, the implementation of affirmative action and financial aid programs, and the dedicated efforts of many individuals transformed the medical student population into what has been in recent years the most demographically and physically diverse group of students ever seen. The entering class of 2001 was composed of 48 percent women and 34 percent minorities, of which 11 percent were underrepresented minorities (African American, Native American, Mexican American/Chicano, mainland Puerto Rican).[7] These statistics, however, do not yet reflect parity with national population demographics.

Although diversity among medical students has increased in recent years, it has not always been, nor is it always now, an unquestioned stan-

6. On the increase in women medical students, see E. S. More, *Restoring the Balance: Women Physicians and the Profession of Medicine, 1850–1995* (Cambridge: Harvard University Press, 1999), 216–229; and Johnson, *U.S. Medical Students, 1950–2000*, 67. On the increase in minority medical students, see Robinson, *AAMC Data Book*, 12–13.

7. For data describing the students who entered medical school in 2001, see "Matriculants by Gender and Race/Ethnicity, 1992–2001," in *AAMC Data*

dard or goal among the powers that be. Some of the individuals who controlled past policies governing the medical educational environment are still working today. In conversations with young medical students, we occasionally hear comments to the effect that discrimination—against blacks or women, for example—no longer exists. But we also hear stories of harassment, humiliation, and rejection directed by classmates or professors against students because of their gender, color, physical disability, or sexual orientation. And we have had such experiences ourselves. We would argue that we are now in a period of transition—medical education has made much progress, but it is still far from where it needs to be.

In Part Three, we include stories from medical students that show how their differences collide with the harsh reality of medical school. How do today's students, with more diverse backgrounds, needs, and views, get along in an educational system that is still largely conformist and traditional in its instructional content, training methods, rules, and rituals? How do today's students deal with either subtle or blatant discrimination? What consequences does discrimination have for their professional options, potential for success, and psychological well-being?

For some, their differences confer added awareness and responsibility to address injustice and suffering. For others, their differences are largely a source of pain, as they encounter prejudice (a Native American man, a black man, and a woman in her surgery clerkship), disadvantages (a fat woman), and unreasonable treatment or refusal to accommodate their needs (a man with chronic back pain, a woman with sickle-cell anemia). Their reactions vary, from articulating specific suggestions for change, to adapting quietly, to finding a special niche or program for themselves. All have tried to make what is arguably a rigid, confining system work for them, to carve their own paths through a thicket of obstacles so that they might one day achieve their dreams.

Warehouse: Applicant Matriculant File (Washington, D.C.: Association of American Medical Colleges, 2002); available online at *http://www.aamc.org/data/facts/famg72002a.htm.*

For each author, the act of sharing his or her story publicly increases awareness and constitutes a step down the road to change. With their diversity and through their self-reflections, we hope that these students will bring new gifts and insights to the practice of medicine and that they might one day play an important role in transforming American medical education into a fairer and more responsive system.

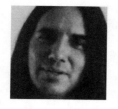

HOKA HEY

I'm a Native American with dark skin and long black hair.

I was told by my chief resident that he thought I would have trouble with my clerkship.

He said that I stand out and that I was under the magnifying glass.

I asked him why.

He thought for a moment and said, "Well, for one thing, you're older."

He also said it must have been difficult for me to leave an Indian community to attend college in a non-Indian community.

He said it must be even more difficult to adjust to medical school and be in a medical community, which is even farther removed from what he suggested was some remote Indian existence.

I never told him that I was born and raised in Los Angeles.

He submitted a failing grade.

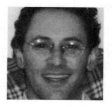

MY NAMES

y name is Tourette Disorder (TD) and Attention Deficit Hyperactivity Disorder (ADHD).[1] TD is a syndrome that can include
motor tics (brief, repetitive movements), vocal tics, ADHD (inat-
tention, disorganization, impulsivity), obsessive-compulsive thoughts
and behaviors (counting, touching, cleaning), and mood disorders (anxiety and depression).

Although I was not formally diagnosed until high school, I have had
tics and symptoms of ADHD since childhood. In elementary school
during the 1970s, I had a strong desire to pick putty out of the window
sill over and over again until it felt right, which resulted in swats from
the principal. I was forced to act on this compulsion to relieve anxiety.
Despite my natural ability as a sprinter in swimming, I developed a
"retropulsion tic" that ended my promising swimming career at the
young age of eleven. Imagine a freestyle sprint competition. Seconds
before touching the wall at the finish, I would encounter an irresistible
need to take several backstrokes, allowing my opponents to glide on to

1. For detailed information about TD and ADHD, see *Diagnostic and Statistical Manual of Mental Disorders*, 4th ed. (Washington, D.C.: American Psychiatric Association, 1994).

victory. During my bar mitzvah, I had to hold inside the most incredible urge to blurt out, "Fuck God," and I unfortunately happened to release it in front of the rabbi while reciting an important prayer. The rabbi never spoke to me again.

As a teenager, I went to a psychiatrist who tried to counsel me against becoming a physician. A straight-A student fascinated by the sciences, I couldn't figure out why my doctor didn't think that medicine was a good career option for me. Sure, I had symptoms that significantly interfered with my activities, but I was still academically successful. Even my mother was concerned about my choice of career, however. "It may be too stressful for you," she often said.

Fortunately, I had a typical case of TD and ADHD. I learned compensatory strategies for my neurodevelopmental problems and studied for long hours in my quiet bedroom after class. As a child, I didn't consciously realize that without reasonable accommodations in school,[2] I couldn't gain much from the primary educational system. My good study habits seemed to teach me what I needed to know, and these skills continued to mature as I progressed through college. And, like most individuals who have TD and ADHD, my tic symptoms diminished during my late teens and in early adulthood. My ADHD, however, continued to plague me, especially when I tried to tackle the increased workload of higher education.

At some point, I realized that having a quiet room and an extended period of time to complete a test greatly improved my performance on exams. In contrast, if I had to race the clock to finish an exam, I noticed myself making significant numbers of careless errors. Before entering medical school, I requested my first official accommodation: extended time on the Medical College Admissions Test (the standardized test

---

2. The term "reasonable accommodations," or "accommodations," refers to some altered condition, such as extended time in which to take an exam, intended to help compensate for a diagnosed disability.

required of all medical school applicants) to help compensate for the effects of my tics and attention problems.[3] I received the requested accommodation and did well on the MCAT and during my medical school interviews.

. . . . .

My name is Chronic Lower Back Pain. While rowing on my university's crew team, I seriously injured my back. The injury led to a lower back pain condition that I couldn't completely rehabilitate in college. I had limited ability to stand or sit for extended periods without experiencing significant pain.

My physician informed me that I would have to "slip through the system" to make it through medical school. I wasn't clear about the meaning of this statement, although I had some idea. For example, I knew that the physical demands of the surgical rotations—long operations that would force me to stand and retract for hours on end—would be virtually impossible to fulfill without some modification in the clerkships. Nonetheless, medical school had been my lifelong dream, and I began my medical education with lots of excitement and optimism as well as some trepidation.

3. One frequent accommodation made for learning-disabled (LD) and/or ADHD students is the provision of extra time to take examinations. Faculty members may believe that this confers an unfair advantage because all students would increase their performance with extended time. But a study found this to be a false assumption. A comparative study of LD and non-LD university students who were matched by their Scholastic Aptitude Test scores were given a reading comprehension test under both timed and untimed conditions. Whereas extra time optimized the performance of the LD students, it did not significantly alter the scores of their non-LD peers. See K. M. Runyan, "The Effect of Extra Time on Reading Comprehension for LD and Non-LD University Students" (paper presented at The Next Step: An Invitational Symposium on Learning Disabilities at Selective Colleges, Boston, November 1989).

Soon thereafter, I began to form a working, trusting relationship with Dr. Smith, the associate dean of student affairs at my medical school. Dr. Smith had been involved with administrative-level academic medicine for more than twenty years. He was highly attuned to disability-related issues and had advocated for many students with disabilities. He expressed a number of important points: First, there was no formal system for individuals who had disabilities. Second, he advised me to ask for more accommodations than I really needed as a bargaining strategy. Third, he cautioned me that, in his experience, academic medicine discriminated against students with disabilities.

My first two years of medical school went relatively smoothly. Then I learned the meaning of "slipping through the system." Before I started my third-year surgical clerkship the head of the department of surgery paged me. In an anxious, quiet voice, he said something along these lines: "Listen, David...you have to be soft with these people. Your letter requesting accommodations is too aggressive, and...please don't tell anyone we had this conversation." Then, in a more sullen tone, he told me that I might fail this rotation. I replied that I thought all the requested accommodations were reasonable, that I understood that the surgery clerkship was run like the military, and that I was aware that I might not be "accepted." Before I knew it, I received a letter stating that the department of surgery could *not* honor my accommodation requests.

I later met with the director of the surgery clerkship, who gave me two options: either completing the clinical part of the rotation without any accommodations or not participating in any of the clinical parts of the clerkship (in other words, I would only attend the lectures and take the exams). But with this latter "special" arrangement, the best grade I could receive was a C. Because I didn't want to appear weak or unmotivated, I told him that I had decided "with great anticipatory anxiety" to participate in the surgical clerkship without any accommodations.

Ironically, I began on the neurosurgical subspecialty and was initially assigned to protracted spinal laminectomy/fusion procedures that were intended to provide pain relief for those who had intractable chronic back pain. I stood through the surgery with a herculean demeanor, held on to that retractor, and engaged in every cognitive pain-reducing strategy known. I lasted about one month. Fortunately, I was not seriously physically injured from the long operations. Once I was "nicely" asked to leave the operating room by the chief neurosurgeon after I broke the sterile field twice—I had a compulsion to touch a cloth that wasn't sterile, which risked introducing infection into the patient. He screamed, "Marcus, what are you doing? If you are going to fuck around, why don't you scrub out for a while!" Later, when I explained my back condition to him and mentioned that my MRI had been read as normal, he sagaciously advised me not to tell anyone else about my back condition.

During my surgical oral exam, I hesitantly explained to the examiners that after one month of the clerkship I had decided to participate only in the lectures and exams. One surgeon who interviewed me seemed to be agitated and was extremely intimidating. At the end of my exam, he let me know—by screaming it at me—that I had failed.

After I failed the clerkship, I went to the director of students in the department of surgery in order to arrange "another attempt to retract successfully" (that is, to repeat the course). He later told me, in effect, "We in the department of surgery do not believe in equal opportunity for students with handicaps, and we will never again make 'special arrangements.' "

.   .   .   .   .

Dr. Smith was my sounding board as I encountered problems getting accommodations. For example, I consulted with him again when the director of students in the department of obstetrics and gynecology hung up on me when I phoned to discuss the possibility of being provided extended time for the final exam. This accommodation was not granted. On the day of the final, after I had rushed through it, believing that I didn't have extra time, the secretary who administered the exam announced that because she was in a good mood she would give everybody additional time.

I spent many sessions with Dr. Smith talking about disability-related issues and relaying stories about faculty members. Some of them were heard making remarks such as "people with disabilities shouldn't be allowed to become doctors," and "students with learning disabilities are slow." We discussed the stereotype of the student with disabilities who makes it through because he or she is "extraordinarily bright, persistent, independent, and hardworking, which compensates for his or her deficiencies." Though this might generally be true, it doesn't negate the need for accommodations.

By my senior year of medical school in 1994, I realized that it might not be a good idea for me to continue to be honest about my disability status. It seemed that my requests for accommodations were not being granted. I began to feel that something was definitely wrong, but I couldn't yet describe the source of my inner conflict. I was aware that physicians took care of many disabled patients. So why was I being treated this way? How could these professors and physicians, our role models, be so ignorant and insensitive? I became aware of an awful feeling of insecurity, shame, and humiliation.

Whatever "slipping through the system" meant, I was not succeeding. During my senior year, an academic hearing committee recommended that I be dismissed from medical school. After seven grueling years of commitment to medicine, it looked as though my medical career was coming to an end. Although I wasn't privy to the conversation during the hearing, I suspected that the committee didn't believe that my disabilities had played a significant role in my surgical clerkships, which I ended up failing twice.

I did have some evidence that the legitimacy of my back condition was questioned. Dr. Smith asked me once about differential diagnoses that I should be exploring, including somatoform disorder (pain disorder), defined as pain that cannot be attributed to a specific physical cause and in which medical test results cannot explain the symptoms. Later, I heard that the committee believed that "psychosocial issues" played a predominant part in my academic difficulties. (I then realized that the biomedical model that necessitates objective evidence for pain definitely has its limitations and can lead to disastrous consequences.) Fortunately, Dr. Smith postponed the delivery of the committee's recommendation to the dean in order to allow me to take a leave of absence for rehabilitation of my back.

That leave turned my life around. I underwent months of intensive physical rehabilitation, which tremendously improved my condition. In addition, I learned about the Americans with Disabilities Act (ADA), a new federal law that provided substantial protections to those with disabilities, including myself. I became involved with the American Medical Student Association's new Task Force on Disabilities (TFD). I attended AMSA's national convention and learned that other students were highly interested in advocacy, education, and modifying the academic medicine environment to aid those with disabilities. The TFD's central mission was to identify and change the problems that have prevented qualified individuals from entering or remaining in the field of medicine. At last I had found others who shared my struggles.

During the TFD's meetings, I heard several optimistic accounts, mainly from Brown University, of educated and dedicated faculty who facilitated the accommodation process for students with disabilities. I also took note of several horror stories. One was about a dean who threatened to expel a deaf medical student if she took her story to the media. Apparently, she had requested an American Sign Language interpreter for her basic science courses, but the school had refused to pay for it, a clear violation of the ADA. Whereas before I had had merely a vague feeling that something was wrong, I now knew that the denial of my requested accommodations may have been in direct violation of federal law.

Though the TFD members had common goals, we were a heterogeneous group because of the hundreds, if not thousands, of types of disabilities. I began seeing many similarities between our new TFD and the advocacy ideology and diversity of AMSA's Lesbian, Gay, and Bisexual People in Medicine. I read articles that highlighted some "minority" concerns, which included issues specific to race, culture, gender, sexual orientation, disabilities, socioeconomic status, and foreign medical students. These articles supported progressive change within the medical school curriculum, improvement of patient care (for example, teaching cultural competency and learning sensitivity to human diversity), and attention to the health and well-being of medical students.

As a result of my newfound knowledge, I wrote a monograph outlining a policy for managing disabled medical students within the medical education system. My exposition recommended that academic medicine develop an affirmative action policy for individuals with disabilities. I reviewed my university's policy for compliance with the ADA and suggested amendments. The monograph was consistent with the ideology of the President's Committee on Employment of People with Disabilities, which included expanded outreach, recruitment, mentoring, training, management, development, and other endeavors designed to help employers hire, retain, and advance qualified workers with disabilities.

. . . . .

I was now able to return to medical school with increased confidence that I truly belonged there. I returned to find that Dr. Smith, who had disagreed with the recommendation to dismiss me from medical school, had advocated on my behalf and influenced the dean to override the committee's decision. I was later informed that this was a very rare event. I was allowed to repeat the surgical clerkships and did so successfully, and I graduated.

Although my condition had improved sufficiently during my physical rehabilitation program so that I could endure the physical demands of the surgical clerkships, I didn't become pain free until I made an important discovery. My most significant treatment modality turned out to be a left foot pedal. Driving with my left foot didn't exacerbate my back condition and helped me to finally eradicate my pain. This one small change in my environment allowed me to succeed both academically and occupationally.

Why didn't any of the "expert" physicians prescribe effective interventions earlier? Should I have expected them to? Looking back now, I see that I initially lacked the knowledge and skills to navigate an environment that was, and continues to be, bureaucratic and inflexible. Who was supposed to facilitate this process and teach me the art of approaching a professor or supervisor/employer to propose necessary accommodations? Who was supposed to advise me of my ADA rights, workable disclosure strategies, and the essential functions needed to become a physician? Who was supposed to help assess the need for specific academic or job accommodations, negotiate the workplace culture, and locate peer role modeling and support? And what would have happened to me had I not met Dr. Smith?

I am fortunate to have successfully overcome the most physically and psychologically traumatic period in my life. Had I not injured my back in college, I probably would have continued to progress satisfactorily in spite of my TD and ADHD. However, I probably wouldn't have educated myself about one of the most important civil rights movements of the new millennium. Neither would I have developed the insight and knowledge about occupational illness and disability management that I now use in my daily work. I still have Tourette disorder, attention deficit hyperactivity disorder, and a history of chronic lower back pain. Although we can assign labels to classify and categorize human differences, I hope that the names I've used are seen as just a small part—albeit an important part—of who I am and what I have become. And, through my journey, I've earned another name: Doctor.

TISTA GHOSH

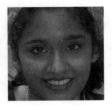

A CASE PRESENTATION

This story is written in the form of a "SOAP" note, an acronym denoting the components of a standard medical record used for writing and documenting a patient encounter. The subjective (S) portion of the record describes what the patient reports as his or her medical problem. Next, all objective (O) findings, such as vital signs and the physical exam, are recorded. The assessment (A) is the interpretation of the subjective and objective findings, which leads the medical care provider to a list of potential diagnoses. Finally, in the plan (P), a course of action is set out, including the treatments given (for example, wound care) or prescribed (medications), other diagnostic studies that may be necessary now or in the future (such as x-rays), and a follow-up contingency schedule (for instance, "return in two days if no improvement").

1/8/99, 06:30

SUBJECTIVE: Twenty-four-year-old woman presents on her first day of surgery rotation with complaints of anxiety, agitation, and apprehension

OBJECTIVE: VS (vital signs): afebrile, tachycardic[1]

Gen (general): well-nourished woman, no acute distress

HEENT (head, ears, eyes, nose, throat): pupils

---

1. The individual is described as not febrile (not having a fever) and experiencing a fast heart rate.

dilated bilaterally, round and reactive to light,
mucous membranes slightly dry
Cor (heart): tachycardic, no murmurs appreciated[2]
Abd (abdomen): hypoactive bowel sounds
Extrem (extremities): diaphoretic[3]

ASSESSMENT: I had heard all about this guy. Dr. Snead, one of the top dogs in the surgery department, was notorious for both his bark and his bite when it came to medical students. His temper, his mood swings, and his chauvinism had reached legendary heights in our medical school. But rumor had it that he was starting to mellow out as he approached retirement, and his last few groups of students had escaped the rotation relatively unscathed.

"It won't be that bad," I reassured my racing heart and my sweaty palms as his massive figure approached. He stopped in front of our group of students, which consisted of three men and me. He scrutinized each of us one by one, his face hard and devoid of emotion.

"You! Stand up straight! This is a hospital, not your mom's couch!" he barked at the first student.

"And you, what the heck is that pocket book you're carrying around? That book is a piece of crap! Next time I see you, I want a real surgery text in your hands. Got it?" I felt my face getting hotter as he turned to gaze at me.

"What's the matter, honey? You nervous?" A sarcastic smile played on his lips. "The rest of you, follow your resident to the wards. But you, sweetheart, you're coming with me. We're going to the OR . . ."

1/8/99, 07:15

SUBJECTIVE: Twenty-four-year-old woman presents to the operating room with complaints of uneasiness, foreboding, and a sense of panic

2. Murmurs are heart sounds that may suggest pathology.
3. Perspiration is noted.

OBJECTIVE: VS: afebrile, tachycardic, tachypneic[4]
Gen: anxious-appearing woman
HEENT: no change from previous exam
Lungs: clear to auscultation bilaterally[5] with notable
shallow respirations
Skin: clammy, diaphoretic

ASSESSMENT: I shouldn't be so anxious about this, I told myself as I meticulously scrubbed my hands outside the OR. I had seen plenty of surgeries during my obstetrics and gynecology rotation. I was not at all unfamiliar with the OR. It was just that this guy was so intimidating! I was worried that he'd blow up at me if I made even the slightest mistake.

And why was he calling me "honey"? Was I somehow projecting the wrong kind of image? Maybe I should have worn my glasses and tried to look smarter. And then I admonished myself. Why should I have to change the way I look? I should be judged on my abilities, my patient skills, and my knowledge base. My thoughts were interrupted by the looming figure standing next to me.

"Let's go, sweetie, let's get this show on the road!" Dr. Snead's voice dripped with impatience, as I followed him into the OR.

1/8/99, 14:30

SUBJECTIVE: Twenty-four-year-old woman presents with complaints of goose-bumps, chills, mental numbness, thirst, and aching feet
OBJECTIVE: VS: tachycardic, hypotensive[6]
Gen: fatigued-appearing, bleary-eyed woman

4. In addition to having no fever and a fast heart rate, the individual is breathing at a very rapid rate.
5. The lung sounds are normal.
6. The individual has a rapid heart rate and low blood pressure, suggesting dehydration.

HEENT: slightly diminished visual acuity, mucous
membranes dry
Lungs: clear to auscultation, excessive sighing noted
Extrem: 1+ lower extremity edema[7]
Skin: mild pallor
MSE (mental status exam): mild deficits in attention and
concentration

ASSESSMENT: I'd forgotten how cold it was in the OR. I could feel the hair rising on my arms, while my teeth chattered silently behind my mask. This surgery would never end. It had already been over seven hours, and we didn't seem close to ending. I felt my feet throbbing dully, as I surreptitiously stretched my lower back. I just knew I'd never make it out of this surgery. I imagined a janitor stumbling onto my stiff, frozen corpse sometime in the distant future, when the surgery was finally over.

"Are you paying attention? Dammit!" Dr. Snead's angry roar jerked me out of my daydream. It was one of the few times he'd even bothered to acknowledge my presence during the past seven hours. It took me a minute to comprehend that it was me he was talking to, not the resident. "Don't just stand there like an idiot! For God's sake, suction that blood already, honey! This isn't an orgasm, sweetheart, you can't just lie back and enjoy it!" His bellow reverberated through the OR. No one moved or said a word.

"I must be in some kind of movie," I told my numbed brain. "This doesn't happen in real life. Professors don't say that to students, at least not in the 1990s. This has got to be one of those made-for-TV movies. There's no other way to explain it." Silently, I watched my hand reach out and suction the blood. This had to be a joke, a one-time thing. Things would get better, I reassured myself. Or maybe I'd just get used to it.

7. Swelling of the feet is noted.

2/4/99, 05:00

SUBJECTIVE: Twenty-four-year-old woman presents with a history of nausea, fatigue, and tension headaches since the onset of her surgery rotation

OBJECTIVE: VS: stable
Gen: thin, haggard-appearing woman
HEENT: diffuse tenderness to palpation in frontotemporal areas[8]
Cor: regular rate and rhythm[9]
Lungs: clear to auscultation, poor inspiratory effort
Abd: mild, diffuse tenderness to palpation, hyperactive bowel sounds, no rebound, no guarding, no masses[10]
Extrem: 2+ lower extremity edema, mild tenderness to palpation of plantar surfaces[11]
MSE: mood depressed with blunted affect, mild to moderate deficits in concentration and memory

ASSESSMENT: I felt like I was always walking on eggshells. No matter what I did, Dr. Snead blew up at me. Weeks had passed, and the sight of him still made my stomach queasy. He had started to warm up to the males on my team, and it was clear they'd all formed a Big Boys Club that I was not invited to join. Dr. Snead graciously let me know, however, that if he and "his boys" ever made a beer commercial with topless scrub nurses, he'd let me participate. I'd make a great nurse, he told me. My male classmates never disagreed.

8. The areas around the temples are tender to the touch.
9. Heart sounds are normal.
10. The stomach hurts and is making loud sounds, but no other stomach abnormalities are found.
11. Both lower legs are swollen, and the soles of the feet are tender to the touch.

Rounds with him had become a daily nightmare. My neck and shoulders were knots of tension by the time they ended. Every day, he fired questions at us mercilessly. Nobody, not even "his boys," dared to miss an answer. I read for hours every night, absorbing the latest articles on the symptoms, causes, and cutting-edge treatments of diseases. I really shouldn't have bothered. Whenever I was next in line to answer a question, his face would take on a patronizing sneer.

"That one might be too hard for you, sweetheart. Why don't we let John answer?"

Every evening, I went home with my head pounding and my stomach churning. Those were some of the worst months in my life. How could one man make me feel so horrible? I was worried about passing, I was scared that I wasn't learning, and, most of all, I was horrified at myself for putting up with Dr. Snead's blatant misogyny. Whenever I'd read in history classes about the treatment of women, I scoffed, wondering why the women didn't just stand up for themselves. And here I was in the late 1990s, silently taking it, just like all the women I'd read about. Maybe I was in shock. After all, I'd never imagined that this type of behavior really existed in the United States anymore, not outside of television. Maybe I was just naïve. And maybe, just maybe, I was too scared to do anything about it. After all, he was one of the heavyweights of the surgery department . . .

ASSESSMENT: Twenty-four-year-old woman rotating through surgery who suffers from . . .

Suffers from what? I wasn't sure, exactly. So many words float through the media today, haunting our thoughts and actions—sexual discrimination, sexual harassment, sexual misconduct . . . the list goes on and on. What does it all mean? Did those words apply to me? All I knew was that I didn't want them to apply. I didn't want to be associated with those terms at all. I just wanted to forget and move on. After all, I was a medical student—my purpose in life was to learn, not to make waves.

And the issues were far too unsettling. No medical student should have to dwell on them.

My perception of medical school had changed dramatically. I felt myself grow hardened and jaded about the so-called learning experience of clinical rotations. Did fear, discomfort, and intimidation really enhance a student's educational environment? Apparently they're supposed to, I often thought cynically.

PLAN: None. I really didn't know what to do. Every night, I weighed my options. I wanted to be brave and address the issue, to be strong and stand up to the system. But the truth was, I didn't have the energy to face the potential consequences. So I adopted the only plan that I felt I could handle: pass the surgery rotation. Keep quiet, get out, and never look back. That was all I had to do.

UGO A. EZENKWELE

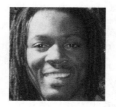

UROLOGY BLUES

I t began as a good day. The sun was just peeking over the buildings, and already I could feel the cool breeze of early fall as it made its way through the house. Just the day before, I had learned that I had received honors for my performance in my internal medicine clerkship, one of the most important and difficult clinical requirements in medical school. Months of hard work had finally paid off. My last major hurdle was the surgery clerkship; after that, the worst of medical school would be over. Just last month, I had obtained a degree in public health, ensuring that when I graduated from medical school I would become one of those professionals whose name is followed by an alphabet soup of letters. Imagine that! A status symbol of knowledge and hard work, those letters would entitle me to respect from my patients and colleagues.

My surgery clerkship was starting today. It consisted of both inpatient and outpatient (ambulatory) surgery. I had been assigned to start with ambulatory surgery clinic, which was an easier way to ease into the hell of surgery. Those less fortunate medical students who were to begin with inpatient surgery had already been in the hospital since before dawn. For the next month, they would be expected to work many more hours than I was, often late into the night, often without sleep and without days off. I, on the other hand, had had a full night's sleep, and I felt prepared and ready to tackle anything. I got out of bed, ate a quick breakfast, and donned my short white coat, which displayed my lowly student status to all those in the field of medicine. I left the house, gave a high five to my buddy two doors down, and dashed to the corner to catch my bus. I was on my way.

At the hospital, as I sat among my fellow students waiting for our ambulatory surgery assignments, we talked anxiously about the long days and nights that we expected over the next couple of months. After what seemed like an eternity, the surgery course director arrived. I was paired up with another student, a fellow from Kansas, to work in the outpatient urology clinic.

Brad was tall and clean-cut, with blue eyes and blond hair—the quintessential all-American male. He had confided in me more than once that he had never known or interacted with any African Americans before he entered medical school. Brad came from a very small town where everyone knew one another. His high school and college experiences had taken place among people with similar backgrounds, interests, and phenotypic makeup. In fact, he often told the story of how, just before he left for medical school, his town had welcomed its first Asian, a Chinese American woman from San Francisco. She had recently married his uncle and had become the yardstick by which all other Asians were measured. Brad recounted with glee how the townsfolk nicknamed her "Connie Chung," after the news personality, much to her chagrin.

Brad's folks, perhaps through no fault of their own, had kept him sheltered. Based on what he saw on television, Brad assumed that all African Americans were athletes, entertainers, drug dealers, or prison inmates. He had heard about the Reverend Martin Luther King Jr., whom he vaguely associated with "civil rights." To him, Malcolm X and Minister Louis Farrakhan were the same type of militants, not to be taken seriously.

Brad's father and grandfather were alumni of our medical school, and he was following a long family tradition. He came to medical school armed with the knowledge of which specialty—otolaryngology—he would pursue. His father and grandfather were otolaryngologists, and a burgeoning practice awaited his graduation from medical school and board certification from the American Board of Otolaryngology.

In contrast, I hardly knew the differences between the various medical specialties, and I would be the first in my family trained as an allopathic physician. My father was an herbalist and a naturopath, a career he had learned from his father in Africa and then brought with him to the United States. He had a practice involving the application of herbal remedies to common maladies, methods that had been tested by time over centuries of African civilization. Most of his patients could not afford Western therapies and turned to my father to diagnose ailments such as hypertension and the flu and to treat them using roots, barks, and leaves. My father knew the limitations of his practice and knew when to refer patients to Western physicians. Although he was well respected among his patients, most others criticized him and labeled his practice as "quack" medicine. They believed that a lack of herbal therapy standardization or rigorous Western research protocols to study these therapies made his practice improper. Medical insurers would never reimburse his services. He had a day job as an economist in order to sustain his family and practiced his brand of medicine on the side. He knew that I would carry on his legacy of healing but that I would not be subjected to the same obstacles he had faced.

As I stood there thinking about my upcoming partnership with Brad, I wondered what it would be like to be paired with someone with whom I seemed to have nothing in common. I had noticed that with other medical students who were different from me, our only conversation would involve medicine or gossip—or perhaps nothing at all—and I worried that Brad and I would fall into that pattern. I knew that my best chance for doing well in surgery would involve having a partner that I could trust. What would I do during those times of uncertainty when the only person I could turn to would be Brad? Could I rely on him for help? How much would we extend ourselves to help each other? Would I jump in with an answer when Brad was being "pimped"—that is, assaulted with a rapid-fire series of questions designed to test his knowledge and humiliate him if he didn't know the answers? Would he offer to help me when I was "scutted out"—singled out to perform menial tasks like photocopying journal articles or buying food for our surgical team? Success in medical school necessitated bonding with your classmates to carry you through the tough times.

On arriving at the urology clinic, Brad and I were told that we would shadow a urologist who was world-renowned for his work with the prostate gland. He was a faculty member in the urology department and was cited as one of the top urologists in the world. His list of patients—which included kings, princes, presidents, and CEOs—read like a *Who's Who in America and Europe.*

Dr. Urology, a small man with a firm handshake and beady, piercing gray eyes, introduced us to his world. Meticulous and precise, he instructed us on our professional appearance and decorum. Our white coats were to be dry-cleaned and starched, not machine- or hand-washed. Our pockets were to contain nothing more than a pen, and our identification badges were to be openly displayed on our lapels—left side only. We were to go into the rooms, introduce ourselves to the patients, obtain pertinent information using templates he had already devised, and present this material to him. He would then enter each room with us, talk to the patient, corroborate our information, grill us on our findings, test us to make sure we had done the necessary readings, and devise a plan of action. He would conduct the infamous rectal examination to assess the prostate gland and then send the patient off for lab tests. For his most important or famous patients, he would conduct the interview himself, and our job was merely to observe.

Once we understood our roles, it was time to perform our duties. Two charts were waiting in the patient bins. I grabbed the first one, and my colleague took the other. We went our separate ways.

I entered the patient's room with a bit of apprehension. I wanted to make a good first impression on both my first urology patient and Dr. Urology. I reminded myself that I was seasoned in the art of patient communication and history taking and that I had done well in my recently completed internal medicine clerkship. The patient was Caucasian, a short and heavyset man. I could see that he was sizing me up.

I smiled, stretched out my hand, and introduced myself. Arms folded, he glared at me, looked away, and cursed under his breath, "What the f—— is this? Who the f—— are you? I don't want to talk to you! I f——ing don't want any affirmative action working on me, let alone a nigger. What the hell is going on? I'm getting the f—— out of here!" With that, he stormed past me through the door and down the hall, all the while swearing and mumbling something about the world being crazy to have let "niggers" into the medical field.

I was floored. As I stood in the doorway, anger, frustration, guilt, and feelings of inadequacy and helplessness coursed through me in a matter of seconds. Years of education, more years of hard work, and numerous degrees had been rendered meaningless. I had done all the right things, volunteered at all the right places, passed all the right exams, represented my family well—and for what? To be called an "affirmative action" and a "nigger"? To have him suggest that I had no right to be here, merely because I'm African American? That there's no possible way any African American could have made it to medical school without affirmative action? That once in medical school all students don't have to fulfill the same requirements, no matter how they were admitted? I knew that he was wrong, but in the face of such blatant hostility, it was hard not to doubt myself just a little.

Then my emotions turned to anger. Why should I, simply because I'm a black man, have to defend myself to him, to myself, or to anyone else? Suddenly, I wanted to give that guy a piece of my mind. How dare he insult me! I was torn between wanting to educate him and knock him on his ass. I wanted him to know about all the accomplishments that people of color had managed to achieve in the face of adversity. I wanted him to know that I had to work twice as hard as my Caucasian classmates so that no one would ever judge me on the basis of my skin color. I wanted to say to him that I was better than he would ever be. I wanted to tell him how ignorant he was. I wanted to yell in his face that I wished he had prostate cancer.

I forced myself to calm down when I saw Dr. Urology coming down the hall toward me, followed by Brad. "What happened?" they asked. After I told them, Dr. Urology took me by the arm and steered me toward one of the empty patient rooms. He apologized for the patient and told me that I should not let this hinder me in any way. He assured me that he was not going to welcome that patient ever again into his office and that he would draft a letter to the dean of students about the entire experience. He apologized again, and I told him I was okay.

I wasn't really okay. Even though Dr. Urology had offered some comforting words, I was upset that the incident had happened at all. Now I felt even more different than I had before, and I didn't believe I could trust anyone enough to reveal my true feelings. I just wanted to make the whole thing go away. Looking at the floor, I quickly stated that this was not the first time I had been judged based on my skin color and it probably wouldn't be the last, but that I could deal with it. Without waiting for a response, I went to grab another chart, knocked on another door, and hesitantly introduced myself to the next patient.

Brad remained quiet and avoided my eyes for the rest of the clinic. At the end of the day, as we walked back to the main medical campus, he confided to me that he was disgusted and upset. He knew about the black-white disparity in America, but he had never seen it firsthand. Back home, his peers and family members had joked about black people in a condescending manner, but he believed they were thinking about the "lazy" ones they had read about or seen on television who were sitting on their porches in the city doing nothing and accepting "free" handouts from the government. It hadn't occurred to him that someone could make similar judgments about me, a hard-working medical student at an elite medical school.

What I really wanted from Brad was automatic understanding and recognition of how I felt—a reaction I likely would have received from another person of color. But I realized that I could use this opportunity to educate Brad about what it's like to be a member of a minority group: to be followed by security guards while shopping in department stores; to be mistaken for an orderly instead of a doctor-in-training; to lack the same access to role models or mentors available to white students. As we talked that afternoon, Brad inadvertently educated me as well, because I had assumed that someone with his background would not be willing to learn about racial discrimination.

Despite what had happened earlier, I guess I could say that that day turned out well after all, but in a way I never would have anticipated. I think Brad and I each became more open to confronting our own racial stereotypes. I gained a new appreciation for Brad, a man with whom I at first believed I had nothing in common.

I still experience incidents of discrimination. Fortunately, because of what happened that day, I am now able to discuss them with my friends and colleagues. After these discussions, all the issues may not be resolved. But having a meaningful exchange of thoughts is an important step in the right direction.

KAY M. ERDWINN

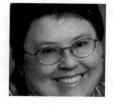

LIKE EVERYONE ELSE

Medical school orientation. I'm elated and terrified at the same time. I sit down on a chair in the lecture hall, distracted by momentary gratitude that it's the kind that pulls away from the table, not one of those "all-in-one" student desks. Then, like everyone else, I listen with half an ear to the dean's speech. What I'm really doing is checking out the other people in my new class. I look around and catalog people shamelessly: she's a science nerd, he's here to make lots of money, he looks genuine, she could be a friend, but him—oh, Gods!—and that one, she looks so boring I doubt I'll even remember her name. And so on. I'm glad we haven't evolved telepathy yet. I'm also noticing the gender, sexual orientation, and racial mixes. I like a group with lots of variety.

I also like to think that I add some variety to a group. Not just because I'm a choral conductor, a cat lover, a yoga teacher, and a juggler, but because of something way more basic: I'm fat. Not just "plus-size," as fashion magazines euphemize, implying, "size 14, 16, 18..." (as if that's fat!). No, I'm "obese," as all the medical journals decree, implying, "about to croak from living an unhealthy lifestyle." Never mind that I exercise regularly, eat reasonably, don't drink, don't smoke, and always wear my seatbelt, even though it's made for—you guessed it—"normal-size" people.

So I'm checking out my new class, seeing who's who, just like everyone else. But unlike everyone else, I have two extra agenda items. The first is the same as in any new situation: to appear indifferent to the stares of those who are Sizing Me Up. The second is, of course, to ascertain if there is Anyone Else. I realize that I'm holding my breath as I scan the room. Are any other fat people here? My eyes land on one man, a cheerful-looking Latino. Well, one, sort of. Stocky, though, not really fat. I sigh, reminding myself that I expected this. The higher my educational level, the fewer fat people I've seen per class. Fascinating trend.

In fact, I was surprised when they let me into medical school. After all, everyone "knows" you can't be healthy and fat at the same time, and I'd expected that fat people might be excluded because they tarnish the "doctor as role model of perfect health" image that the medical profession would like to maintain. But the University of California at Davis admitted me without a single comment on the subject from anyone, at least in my hearing. It was great to beat the odds and make it into med school. Nicer still not to be forced to deal with ignorant interviewers who assume that I have an eating disorder, a rotten relationship with my mother, a fear of men and sex, poor self-esteem, or any of the myriad physical diseases fat people are supposed to be susceptible to.

So, it looks like I'm the only fat person in a med school class of one hundred. According to the statistics, there should be others like me in my class. Where are they? Some were probably denied admission because their interviewers couldn't see past their size. But many more who are smart and talented enough are probably caught in the trap of using their time, energy, and money trying futilely to lose weight rather than accomplish a meaningful goal in life. They believe that something's wrong with their character, appearance, and worthiness because they're fat, and they put all their efforts into trying to correct the supposed defect. I feel sorry for them, especially since I was one of them twelve years ago. No more. I'm here, achieving my dream to be a physician. But even I don't weigh enough to fill the empty space where those other fat people should be.

. . . . .

Gross anatomy lab. Aptly named. Like everyone else, I'm both revolted and fascinated. Unlike everyone else, I have to stand on a plastic foot-stool to see. Other short people (I'm five feet two inches) who are of average size can manage without a stool, but if I lean over—as they do—to see, I have to come into contact with the cadaver and formalin, because I can't suck in my beautiful round abdomen enough to avoid it.

Is this a big deal? It sure is. You see, the formalin and bits of tissue escape from our less-than-pristine dissection efforts, cover the floor and my stool, and make it treacherously slick. Everyone has to be careful, but because I get up and down umpteen times an hour, I slip and fall several times. This is embarrassing, occasionally painful, and, most of all, unnecessary. If the medical school would realize that we don't all have the physical proportions of Dr. Kildare, they'd provide dissection tables that are adjustable, or at least stools that are safe. (I had to bring my own Rubbermaid cheapie from home.) One size does not fit all.

. . . . .

Third year. Finally, I'm starting clinical medicine, and, like everyone else, I'm ecstatic to be done with endless lectures, memorizing, and cramming for boards. Unlike everyone else, I'm spending my last couple of vacation days trying to "fit" into life on the wards.

"Hi! What's your largest lab coat size for med students?" I ask, keeping my face cheerful, despite the obvious discomfort of the hospital laundry clerk. All the Gods forfend that a fat person should take care of herself so forthrightly.

As I expected, after a bit of half-hearted rummaging, the clerk names a number two sizes too small. I thank her with my jolly mask still in place and turn away, letting my anger show as soon as my back is turned. It's not the clerk's fault, but it really hurts that all the average and small people are guaranteed a lab coat, and fat people aren't.

I grind my teeth as I make my way to the operating room changing area. I riffle through the scrubs, trying not to be too obvious. This time, the largest size is three sizes too small. I restrain myself from dumping the lot of them on the floor; childish retaliation is entertaining in fantasy but not very useful in real life.

Fortunately, I was an excellent Girl Scout (although I never got to wear the uniforms; they didn't come in my size), so I'm prepared. I've already found the one store in Sacramento where I can buy lab coats and scrubs, and I know from experience that I could also go online or get a catalog from a couple of companies. I'll manage; I always do. So I show up on my first day of surgery rotation with fancy new scrubs. I had to buy them myself, and I paid over half again what the average sizes in the same styles cost. I was told by the sales clerk that the price difference was based on the extra material used. Does an extra yard of simple cotton-polyester fabric really cost twenty dollars?

. . . . .

Life on the wards is hard for everyone. Even though learning to work as a doctor is a genuine privilege, the hours are grueling. Like everyone else, I'm less than thrilled about working until I can no longer see straight, let alone provide thoughtful and empathic medical care. Unlike everyone else, I'm in real trouble physically. I practice yoga and walk daily, but I'm hardly an athlete. The doctors I work with are mostly in their late twenties (I'm ten years older), average size or thin, and taller than five foot nine. Clearly they are Dr. Kildare clones, risen from a celluloid grave.

The clones think nothing about running up four flights of stairs or "walking" across the hospital campus so fast that I literally have to jog to keep up. (Actually, the normal-size women on my teams have the same problem; our legs are just shorter.) And it's nothing for the clones to stand in the hallways for three hours on rounds. They don't think to ask a lowly med student whether she's able to do any of this. Real physicians can do everything, you see, and we never, ever complain or take care of ourselves if it means doing things differently than the rest of the team. Lemmings of the world, unite!

Nonetheless, I've become quite adept at volunteering to put the charts back and meeting the team on the next floor; that way, I can go upstairs at my own pace or, on a bad day, take the elevator. I also blatantly sit down during rounds whenever possible. Plantar fasciitis, a repetitive motion injury that causes chronic heel pain, makes standing for long periods pure torture for me. I get lots of furtive disapproving looks, but too bad. I have to take care of myself. Fortunately, my work is good enough that no one can rag on me for not going with the unspoken behavioral program. And, oh, does that annoy them! Even though it's hard to swim against the current, I do confess to some unholy glee at their discomfiture. It almost makes up for the pain.

Anyway, it's stupid to think that being able to run upstairs or stand around for hours will make me a better doc. It's simply part of the traditional hazing of the physician-in-training. I'd like to give them all 150-pound packs and watch them run up four flights of stairs. Then I'd float serenely from the elevator, with my white coat miraculously transformed into wings and a halo. With a beneficent smile, I'd cluck sympathetically as they collapsed on the floor, wheezing. Then I'd save them all from respiratory failure by administering 100 percent oxygen, and they'd be forever in my debt. In gratitude, they'd decree a maximum sixty-hour work week, seated rounds, and a sane walking pace. They'd build a statue of me in the front courtyard, and...Hmmm. Time to return to reality. If they were that grateful, they'd probably name some loathsome disease after me. Yuck.

· · · · ·

It's amazing how some of the docs talk about their patients. No one is spared, of course, but they really ream the fat patients behind their backs:

"She's fat on the outside and fat on the inside!"

"There isn't anything we can do for her until she stops shoveling the food in her mouth!"

"He's just a 'Blue Bloater' " (someone with chronic bronchitis).

"It's so goddamned hard to operate on these fat ones—why do I bother?"

"She needs Jenny Craig more than she needs a doctor."

And on and on and forever on. The worst part is how oblivious they are, these sterling representatives of compassionate healing and scientific rationality. They seem unaware of much of the medical research over the past twenty-odd years, so their general assumption is, "Fat people are fat because they eat too much—period. If they wanted to be thin, they could just go on a diet. But they're too gluttonous, weak-willed, and self-hating to do that."

These medical "experts" don't seem to know that most people who diet don't succeed. (My opinion: Diets don't work and are probably harmful, so it's bad medicine to prescribe them. *Primum non nocere*, and all that.) In one study in Denmark, for example, by the five-year mark after dieting, only 3 percent of participants had kept off even half the weight they had lost. Likewise, only 16 percent had done so after gastroplasty (stomach stapling).[1] So much for "just going on a diet."

Also, most fat people aren't always gluttonous; they don't eat significantly more than most normal-size people. A study reported in the *International Journal of Obesity* couldn't find any difference in eating habits based on size, though it did find some based on dieting history.[2] (People—fat or not—tend to binge in response to food restriction.)

The doctors I'm training with have taught me that fat people with heart disease should lose weight. Nathan and Robert Pritikin and Dean Ornish have doubtless made millions on this medical "wisdom." The

1. For information about the Danish study, see F. M. Berg, ed., *Obesity and Health*, May 1989, 33–38.

2. K. S. Kissileff, H. A. Jordan, and L. S. Levitz, "Eating Habits of Obese and Normal Weight Humans," *International Journal of Obesity* 2 (1978): 379.

trouble is, no one has ever mentioned that a famous post–World War II study by Keys et al. discovered that food restriction has severe effects on the heart. In this study, healthy, normal-size young men were put on a 1,500- to 1,600-calorie a day diet for several months. They lost an average of 20 percent of their cardiac muscle mass, and their cardiac output was decreased by an average of 50 percent.[3] It seems dangerous, therefore, to make people who are already "heart-stressed" go on a diet.

And what about fat people being weak-willed? The diet in Keys's study was sensible, according to popular wisdom. The volunteers, all fit and lean young men who seemingly had an abundance of will power (they were a group of conscientious objectors who had opposed World War II) couldn't hack it. They became depressed, anxious, and lethargic; and they started obsessing about food, wanting to steal it and eat in secret.[4] In short, they acted like people with eating disorders—the same way my stalwart teachers claim that fat people act. (Maybe some fat people do so because they're dieting, not because they have an eating disorder.) Anyway, despite the extreme discomfort of living with food restriction, many fat people have the will power to try much more stringent diets than the lads in the Keys study—over and over again. Weak-willed? Right.

So the good doctors seem to view fat people in much the same way the general populace does, despite some evidence to the contrary. They want fat people to starve themselves, take dangerous pills, get their stomachs stapled, and, best of all, join a gym and endure smug looks and outright taunts, just to become like all those thin, stylish, and judgmental people in their designer aerobic outfits.

I remember going to a physician for foot pain during my pre-med years. He opened the door to the exam room, took my chart from the

3. The Keys study is described in F. M. Berg, ed., *Obesity and Health*, January/February 1993, 8–11.

4. For information about the behavior changes recorded in the Keys study, see W. Bennett and J. Gurin, *The Dieter's Dilemma* (New York: HarperCollins, 1982), 11–16.

slot on the door, and, without opening it, looked at me and said, "I know what's wrong with you—you need a reducing diet!"

I felt my gut tighten in fury, but I answered mildly, "Perhaps you'd like to check what the chief complaint is before deciding that."

He was royally offended and refused to examine me or order an x-ray. In the car after my appointment, I cried in rage and humiliation for half an hour. All part of going to the doc. Then I tossed his card in the trash and switched to more supportive shoes, which fortunately solved my problem.

To be fair, I need to admit that some docs are starting to understand that eating reasonably and being physically active are more important than one's number on the scale. And it's certainly true that some fat people really do eat compulsively or are couch potatoes. But not all of us. And plenty of thin people fit that description too.

Most of all, though, fat prejudice is a case of "blaming the victim," because the assumption is that being fat is a matter of choice—as if anyone would choose to endure daily hostility and, even worse, the well-meaning strangers who intrude with comments such as, "You should try Herbalife, dear. It really works, and you have such a pretty face—it's a shame to let yourself go like this." (This really happened to me.) And, of course, we prefer to put up with the clothes and the restaurant, theater, and airplane seats that don't fit us; the magazines that promise miracle cures to "melt away that ugly fat"; and the TV shows and movies that cast us as bingeing buffoons. All because we're too stubborn, too weak, or too neurotic to suffer a little in order to join the ranks of the good, healthy people. As if.

·   ·   ·   ·   ·

Back in med school, it's time for orthopedics. Not my favorite specialty. Still, I'm here to learn, and like everyone else, I make the best of the rotations that I'm less interested in. Unlike everyone else, I'm dealing with some of the fallout from the glib assumptions made by the "orthopods" (the orthopedists).

For example, one of my patients is a woman of about two hundred pounds who is five foot six. The doctor sweeps in, glances at the chart, and tells her that if she went on a diet of 1,000 calories per day, the pain in her knees would be gone. Poof! Like thin people never get osteoarthritis. They do, and they get treatment, not write-offs like "go on a diet." Fortunately, this is a savvy woman. When the doc leaves in a swirl of white-coated self-importance, she looks at me, and we both burst out laughing.

"Who the hell does he think he is?" she snorts.

"Someone who's never been fat and tried to diet," I answer candidly. Our eyes meet in perfect mutual understanding.

It turns out that this woman has been eating extremely carefully and swimming every single day for years. Too bad the doc left before she could tell him that. He might have learned that some fat people really do take care of themselves. Actually, I've learned something, too. From now on, I'm going to take an eating, dieting, and exercise history from every single patient. That's something most doctors don't bother to do, but I think it's the only way to get accurate information about patients. Assuming that we know their habits based on their size clearly doesn't work.

· · · · ·

So now I'm in the home stretch, with four months of medical school to go. Like everyone else, I have a pervasive case of senioritis. Unlike everyone else, I'm still gritting my teeth against the bigotry I experience as a fat person in the narrow-minded culture of medicine. I'm angry, I'm hurt, and some days I'm too damned tired to keep up my defenses, so when I hear some doc's fatophobic comment, my self-esteem does a crash-and-burn. But when all is said and done, I refuse to believe that I'm inferior because I'm fat. In some ways differently-abled, yes, but just like everyone else, I have my good, bad, and indifferent qualities. And I think my fat is one of the indifferent ones. I will not allow self-hatred and rage at others' ignorance to fester in me or to spoil my love for my patients and for myself, a beautiful, competent, compassionate—and fat—physician.

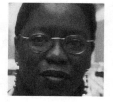

DARING TO BE A DOCTOR

E very time I sign a patient's chart on the ward, I experience a small dilemma, wondering how to identify myself. In addition to my name, I'm supposed to indicate my title. Should I really put *MS* 5/6 after my name, meaning that I am a medical student in my fifth year out of what will be a total of six? I'm afraid that would prompt a lot of questions:

"Why is it taking you six years, and not the regular four, to complete medical school?"

"Are you getting another degree?"

"Did you take time off during medical school?"

"Did you do research?"

I actually have done some research. I could tell them about my work in thalassemia at Stanford and in sickle-cell anemia at Oakland Children's Hospital. I could also tell them about the magazines in which I have been featured as a medical student overcoming personal obstacles. I definitely have accomplished enough to explain away at least one year.

But beneath any explanation I choose to give lies a more personal truth that I do not want to reveal to my colleagues. I have sickle-cell anemia, a blood variant that helps to protect against malaria but that also causes oxygen-carrying red blood cells to change shape (to sickle) and thereby lose their ability to sustain bones and vital organs, such as the spleen, liver, and lungs, with needed oxygen. And, to my dismay, it has taken a turn for the worse in the past two years.

I don't want to explain that I kept getting sick and had to take time off, extending my third year of medical school into two. I don't want them to think that I'm not a hard worker. I'm well aware of the stereotypes of minorities and women in medicine. Yet, in my heart, I know that I have worked extremely hard, considering that I am succeeding in medical school while in constant bone pain and on a host of medications, all with undesirable side effects. I mean, try having to decide whether to live in pain or to live in constant heavy sedation from your pain medications.

Last year, I had four lung infarctions, in which the blood supply to my lungs was inadequate, causing indescribable pain. I also had a transient ischemic attack (a ministroke), in which there wasn't enough blood supply to my brain. And, as a result of all my recent symptoms, my doctors made a big push to screen me as a possible candidate for a bone marrow transplant. Yeah, what a slacker I was in my fourth year (of six). For the moment, I'm tempted to lie and write *MS 3/4*. In my heart, however, I know that I should write the truth, because it is the truth.

In all fairness, I know that there are humane, compassionate doctors in the medical field, many of whom may be my colleagues and who would understand my situation. There are even doctors who probably identify with my challenges and who would wholeheartedly support my lifelong dream of becoming a doctor, which began when I was a child growing up in South America. And there are those who believe in never giving up hope, who believe that when life serves you lemons, you make lemonade, lemon tart, lemon drops, and lemon chess pie.

But there are also cynics along every path, and I have been amazed to see that even "educated" doctors could become annoyed at me for having a genetic disease and choosing to enter the field of medicine. These people have made it hard to ask for accommodations for any aspect of my disability. And, frankly, if I ever saw any way to wing it, even with consequences to my health, I usually did it without asking for a single thing.

One night, for example, I asked the attending physician, who is in charge of the medical team, if I could please be on call from home after 2:00 A.M. I had been experiencing severe sickling in my lungs, which felt like constant, deep, stabbing pains that I can only describe as slow torture. If untreated, these episodes usually result in permanent damage to my lungs. This particular episode had started quite suddenly on my call day (a "work day" in which I was expected to put in a full day of work, stay through the night, and continuously work the following full day). But, by some stroke of luck, I had admitted my maximum number of patients for the night, and they were all stabilized and doing well. "I live just down the street, Dr. Green. I could be here in minutes if anyone paged me." I told him about my situation and explained that the huge oxygen tank I needed for my lung treatment was stationed at home.

"Well, Simone, I'm sure that's okay, but I do think you're depriving yourself of the total medical student experience. All of your colleagues stay the night. What are you planning to do if this problem continues? I mean, if this is too hard for you, what will you do during residency?"

I was quite embarrassed. I wanted to say that this didn't happen often and that I would be better soon. I wanted to say that I didn't think my colleagues would stay if their lungs were collapsing, as mine were. I wanted to say many other things. But, as I looked in the face of this young attending, I realized that he had probably never had a time when he was sick. He might never have been hospitalized for anything. He probably assumed that he somehow deserved his good health. My poor health, for the moment, was an inconvenience to him, never mind me. At that moment, I realized that it is not my disease that breaks my spirit, but the people I have to fight every day who won't give me a chance to live in spite of my disease.

The hardest thing I have had to do as a medical student is to go to the emergency room to be treated by my colleagues. If I ever go to the ER, it's usually as a last resort. It can happen because nothing at home is working to alleviate my painful episodes, or because I am having some complication with my lungs and I know that the wisest thing is to turn myself in. And I dread it. But I know that I must go, and it's the only ER anywhere close to my house. I'm always a little shy at first when a medical student walks in to take my history, especially if I know or even recognize him or her as one of my colleagues. There is always an awkward interchange: "Oh! I'm so sorry you're here! What clerkship are you doing now? Oh, don't worry, they'll understand...yeah. You know what, let me go and get a resident..."

I always feel bad for the both of us, really.

Then comes the time when I have to give my history from scratch. I do so in an orderly and precise manner, since I am a medical student and all. And because I am a medical student, I should definitely be answering questions phrased in complex medical terminology.

"Why don't you give me your H&P, Simone?" the doctor asks, referring to a history and physical.

As I look up at the doctor, while my pain is so intense I feel like there's heat coming out of my ears, the last thing I want to do is make a formal presentation.

During the worst days of that bad year, what kept me going was the support of those around me. For instance, my husband, who has been my biggest advocate, never forgot to remind me of my college days, when I was told: "Simone, why are you applying to these out-of-reach schools, where other people have such a slim chance of getting in?" I would just shrug and say, "I think I'll still keep them on my list. After all, the worst they can say is no, and I've certainly heard that before!" As my husband reminded me, I could recall these events as water under the many bridges I've had to cross.

I also had my "fair *and* foul weather friends." They were my "4:00 A.M. when I'm having a painful crisis episode and need to go to the ER" friends. They were my "I'll bring you dinner for the next two weeks so you can get back on your feet" friends. They were my "the heat went off at church so I brought you an extra jacket to stay warm in service" friends. And, yes, they were my "party hearty and healthy" friends. And they came in all sizes, shapes, and colors. This group of friends, day by day, without knowing it or taking any credit, enriched my life with a dimension that had nothing to do with school and yet had everything to do with it.

My pain and hardship, like sickle-cell disease itself, has also conferred advantages. I have learned to maintain the peace and focus it takes to keep my goals in sight in the face of discouragement. I will always have the priceless gift of knowing what it feels like to be a patient. I know what it feels like to go to work sick—and to take care of the sick. And I know what it feels like to be hospitalized, at the mercy of doctors. And I know what it feels like to be kept alive on a respirator, what it tastes like to have a plastic tube down my throat opening up my lungs, and what it means to wait over time for someone to pronounce my verdict of death or life. But most of all, I know that when my patients walk through the door, they want to be remembered for all the great and many things they can still do despite their diseases, not only for the few things they can't. And I hope that I always remember to cheer them through their disabilities even while accepting their limitations.

If I can step back from my day-to-day problems and remember that I am setting the pace as an African American woman with sickle-cell anemia in medical school, I realize that my dilemma of exactly how to identify myself is indeed a small one. It shouldn't matter whether I write *MS 4/6*, *MS 3/4*, or *MS 5/6*. What ultimately matters is that when I finally walk across the stage at graduation, I will be a physician.

A GRADUATION SPEECH

F amilies, friends, faculty, and staff, the class of 2000 at the University of California at Davis School of Medicine is happy and honored to share our exhilarating and momentous day with you. We want to take this opportunity to share our triumphs and trials over the past few years and to ponder our dreams and hopes and fears as we ready ourselves for the journey ahead.

We began our medical training full of excitement: the excitement of childhood dreams and adult ambitions realized. We had made it into medical school. We knew that we would work hard to become the best doctors. But we were also full of fear. "What if they find out that I am not that smart?" "Wow, John read the entire anatomy syllabus already, and orientation is only half over!" We triumphed when we fully appreciated the different talents in each of us, when we began to feel comfortable and proud of our unique gifts. In the basic sciences years, we mastered strange words such as "tachyphylaxis" and "menometrorrhagia." In the clinical years, we successfully decoded the cryptic go-home signal: "You can go home, if you want to." We learned that "going home" was considered weak, so we stayed. "Farewell, soft fluffy bed. I'll see you in four or five hours."

Over the past few years, we have grown both professionally and personally. Professionally, we matured from thinking that diabetes is just a condition that precludes people from eating too much sugar to learning that diabetes is a disease that affects every single system in the body and then to meeting people with diabetes. We moved from having an idealized desire to help and serve our fellow human beings to providing actual care and compassion as we meticulously checked our patients' feet for diabetic ulcers. We won't soon forget the woman who had no legs, no vision, whose voice was mangled by a recent stroke, struggling to tell us that she needed to be turned.

In our personal lives, we overcame many trials: the deaths of loved ones, new marriages, failed relationships, parenthood, depression, hospitalizations, and academic probations. But our greatest personal triumph is that we survived. We survived difficult, intense, and sometimes dehumanizing medical training and emerged as whole human beings, with our hearts and souls intact. We survived, still ourselves, because we refused to let the one-dimensional curriculum of biochemistry, pathology, pharmacology, and still more science define us. We prevailed in taking time to explore the many sides of our selves that make us human. We allotted time for seeing movies, performing research, running marathons, having babies, obtaining Master of Public Health degrees, organizing American Medical Student Association events, serving on committees, and volunteering. Time for families and friends. Time to reflect, and time to make fun of ourselves as we gathered yearly for our "Mirth Control" talent show and roast.

Our endeavors were more meaningful and less difficult because we had families and friends who cherished and supported us and made sacrifices for us. For these people, we bow our heads in gratitude. Class of 2000, close your eyes and send thanks to all the significant people in your life. We would also like to acknowledge our adopted family here at the UC Davis School of Medicine. We thank the special and rare teachers who called us their colleagues, who treated us with care and respect, who taught us compassion by modeling kindness. We are so proud to be your colleagues. We will miss you!

As we look forward, we dream of the day that all our debts are paid; we hope for three hours of sleep each night, come the beginning of our internships in July; and we fear. We fear that our ideals will turn into cynicism as we become overworked and sleep-deprived. That sick people will become burdens to be discharged from our service. That patients' concerns and vulnerabilities stemming from their illness will become whines to be written off as psychological "Axis II" diagnoses. We fear the prediction of Dr. Howard Spiro, the director of the Program for Humanities in Medicine at Yale, that our hearts will turn to stone as we watch alcohol and drugs destroy lives over and over, while all we can do is patch here and there. We fear that our anguish will fade and our empathy will run dry after repeated encounters with children molested and beaten in body, maimed in spirit, and crippled in emotion. We fear that juggling life's daily toils will cause us to adopt phrases such as "that's reality" and will dishearten our courage to fight for our patients, to serve as agents for change in our community, and to let our ideals guide us.

We fear that we do not possess the wisdom to balance modern technology and ancient folk healing, to integrate Western and Eastern medicine, skills that will be needed in the twenty-first century. We fear that we do not possess the wisdom to take on the paradoxical responsibility of caring for individual humans and caring for humankind. Or the ability to juggle the many roles of a physician: as healer, teacher, technician, fighter, and friend. And how in the world will we be able to care for the complex interplay of our patients' bodies, emotions, and spirits? Perhaps most frightening of all, we fear that we may ultimately be replaced by some slick, imperturbable, and precise artificial intelligence.

To our fears, the Wizard of Oz asserts, "True courage is facing danger when you are afraid." And the Scarecrow points out, "You are wise; it takes great wisdom to follow your heart, to have found time in your jammed medical curriculum to explore your different interests." And the Tin Man cheers, "Your heart is now joyous, celebrating your accomplishments. I see it in your smile." And the Lion roars, "You are courageous to take on the sacred and difficult responsibilities of a physician."

Class of 2000, as you undertake the journey ahead, you will travel through strange lands, where the inhabitants rely on total equanimity. They will advise and persuade you to dispose of your emotions and harden your hearts. Do not be fooled. Remember the classic words of Dr. Francis Weld Peabody in his famous lecture "The Care of the Patient," delivered to Harvard medical students in 1926: "The physician who attempts to take care of a patient while he neglects this [emotional] factor is as unscientific as the investigator who neglects to control all the conditions that may affect his experiment."

Without your heart, you will not feel your patients' anguish and joy. Without your heart, you are replaceable. Let your heart guide you; consult it often in the care of your patients and of yourself. Yes, of yourself. It will turn to stone only if you abandon it. On your journey, you will traverse dark forests where trees bear dollar bills and the beasts have heads of red tape and bodies of corporations. Do not let them weaken your courage. Courage to stand up and fight for what you believe. Courage to think outside the box, to challenge your teachers and your schooling.

Your patients and your students will question your ideas and beliefs. Have the courage to consider those questions. In your personal life, have the courage to recognize cynicism and discontent as signals for change. Have the courage to live life fully and passionately.

On your journey, use your wisdom. Wisdom for knowing when to be conventional, when to be unconventional, and when to be both. Wisdom for knowing when to use logic, when to use intuition, and when to use both. Wisdom for knowing when to look at your patient's MRI, when to see her spirit, and when to view both. Wisdom for knowing when to use common sense and when to toss it to the wind. Wisdom for knowing when to follow the yellow brick road and when to paint it red, blue, or green. Wisdom to change to a new path if it makes your heart sing. Wisdom to measure your success on your own terms as you travel on.

To our fears, I say, "Reality is what you make it!" I leave you with my best wishes, my warmest laughter, and my business card for future referrals. Congratulations class of 2000, and good journey.

EDITORS' NOTE

This graduation speech was never delivered. The University of California at Davis School of Medicine selects its graduation speeches in a competition. Any student who wishes to be considered must write his or her speech and deliver it to a selection committee composed mostly of students. Whoever wins the most votes is selected as the graduation speaker. Thao Nguyen, whose first language is not English, did not win. Nonetheless, we chose to include her speech in this volume because we think it illustrates some of the issues many medical students face.

Like many of the stories in this book, Thao's speech can be construed as a positive portrayal of her medical school experience. It quickly highlights some of the milestones we all faced as we went through medical school and makes us remember certain moments with both pride and relief. Relief, because few, if any, of us, would ever return to endure the hazing we experienced in medical school. Alluding to the lack of sleep with a whimsical "Farewell, soft fluffy bed," makes us laugh, but with an edge of discomfort. Sleepless nights are something that all medical students know. And we all have spent nights on call without sleep as a way of "proving" that we're tough.

But a truly sleepless night has a far more visceral reality than the mere mention of the words. It's almost impossible to convey to someone who hasn't gone through this process what the experience is really like. To be so tired that you obsess about sleep and that all you want is to close your eyes or put your head down, if only for a few minutes. To be ravenous as your body begs for sustenance to keep functioning. To be shivering cold at five in the morning because your cortisol levels are dropping. To feel so weak that you ride the elevator one floor or to be so mentally dulled that you can't construct cohesive sentences. Then, as the next day starts for most, but only continues for you, being verbally harassed or humiliated by attending physicians about why you made certain decisions or why you failed to do something that was out of your control. Exhaustion is never an excuse.

"When I was a medical student thirty years ago, I had to work forty-eight hours straight," says your attending physician. "If you can't work under the most extreme situations, how can you be a good doctor? What's going to happen when you really start to practice medicine and have to make critical decisions without any sleep?"

As the day continues, you grow more tired and doze off whenever you sit down. But you must continue working until all your patient care is completed for that day. The unspoken words condone sleeplessness as acceptable. But working for thirty-six continuous hours is not only inhumane; it's completely unnecessary and detrimental to patients.

In her graduation speech, Thao merely glosses over lack of sleep and other hardships, as most medical students would. But why? Anyone with any sensitivity agrees that such practices are wrong. But standard human responses to extreme situations are to minimize them or make them into jokes. Other responses to some of the dehumanizing events that occur in medical school are to quit, to try to pretend that everything is okay, to turn one's focus inward, to become depressed, to commit suicide, to turn to drugs or alcohol, or to try to change the system. The stories in this book represent some of these responses.

It is a natural human tendency to deny reality or to reconstruct it. We do this to protect our loved ones and ourselves. But this tendency, manifest in the happy endings of many stories in this book, raises larger questions. If we become too successful in our denials and other coping strategies, can we articulate or even see what is really happening? If we can't assess or address bad situations accurately, how can we ever make meaningful changes in our lives or improve the system? How can we really know our capabilities or ourselves?

A further examination of both Thao herself and her speech gives a clearer view of some of the realities of life as a medical student. For instance, Thao mentions overcoming many trials, including depression and academic probation. Readers would never know, however, that Thao herself, a Vietnamese refugee raised in a single-parent household, was placed on academic probation and threatened with expulsion after a bout of depression. Despite these difficulties, she was one of the few students who openly supported other students, by lending them her lecture notes, by listening to their problems, by giving encouragement and helping them study when they had academic difficulties, and by helping student organizations raise money for underserved medical clinics.

These examples demonstrate not only Thao's remarkable generosity but also the urgent need for medical schools to provide more tutorial, counseling, and other support to their students. That any motivated student would be subjected to the humiliation of possible expulsion as the result of a medical illness should be unacceptable. It is too easy to be caught up in the positive tone of Thao's speech and miss its subtleties, to acknowledge the passing of milestones or the tolerance of difficulties but not to consider the actual human emotional consequences behind the words.

Toward the end of her speech, Thao outlines the fears that many medical students face as they ascend into the ranks of interns: the long hours, the lost spirit, and the compromising of patient care. But what some of us really fear is that there are medical students who don't fear these things, because they have not faced the complex reality of their situation or because they have not pushed themselves to look beyond what they've been told to think.

Finally, Thao invokes courage and reminds us that being a doctor takes much more than simply learning the science—it takes heart, commitment, personal sacrifice, self-reflection, and humor. We believe that the stories in this volume convey these traits and more. Our hope is to inspire those who have both the fear and the courage to keep up the struggle and to be honest with themselves and others, because they are the people we want as our colleagues, friends, mentors, and physicians.

AFTERWORD

We cannot end this book without considering some solutions to the problems faced by today's medical students. Although we realize that the struggles within medicine are connected to those of the broader society, the suggestions we offer here focus strictly on improvements within the medical education system. Some of these changes are already taking shape at different medical schools around the country, but we believe that a complete overhaul of the system, based on these ideas, will eventually be necessary to educate those who will become our best doctors.

As we look back at medical school, we see an educational environment that has not kept up with the times, one that continues to be mired in "old school" thinking. It reflects the attitudes of those too proud to admit that a major overhaul is needed and too traditional to make drastic but courageous changes.

One could perhaps argue that our educational system has successfully trained generations of physicians in the past. But these physicians were a homogeneous group, indoctrinated to become infallible figures of science and authority. The demographics of both our nation's population and the group of people who choose to enter the medical profession are changing. Doctors today are less frequently seen as all-powerful; many people advocate a basic change in the doctor-patient relationship, promoting a new ideal of equal partnership with shared responsibility. In addition, economic forces are reshaping the medical profession, resulting in an even more complex role for physicians. Within a system of managed care, for example, the physician enjoys less status, must provide more accountability, and needs to function as a team player. Reflecting these societal changes, many students have different reasons for choosing medicine than the students of the past. Many of today's students are not willing to shed their identities, to be molded into another person's vision of what a doctor should be.

To meet our changing expectations of doctors, we will need to change our medical school admissions policies. We propose that medical schools abolish MCAT testing and minimum grade point averages as criteria for interviews. MCAT scores do not correlate with clinical performance in post–medical school residency training.[1] Not only is the test itself expensive, but the desire to do well causes many students to spend as much as several thousand dollars on test preparation courses and materials. These courses are now so widespread that not taking them is seen as placing an individual at a distinct disadvantage. Minimum grade point average requirements screen out potentially solid candidates who might have encountered academic difficulties because of family commitments, an illness, or the logistics of dealing with a disability. Admissions committees should read all of the applications submitted by those who have met minimum standards such as a college degree and basic science course requirements. Reducing or waiving secondary application fees and conducting interviews by telephone, videoconferencing, or regional meetings could also eliminate significant financial barriers for some medical school applicants.

Reshaping the criteria for selecting medical students may be among the most difficult reforms a medical school could undertake. Although a

1. See R. C. Davidson and E. L. Lewis, "Affirmative Action and Other Special Consideration Admissions at the University of California, Davis, School of Medicine," *Journal of the American Medical Association* 278 (1997): 1153–1158.

comprehensive exploration of this issue is beyond the scope of this discussion, we do support the concept of affirmative action and programs that are intended to increase access to educational opportunities for those who have historically suffered from policies of exclusion. We also believe that a more diverse physician population will better serve the needs of our broader society. Thus far, affirmative action has been the only systematic approach that has even attempted to meet such goals; if affirmative action is struck down in the courts or through public policy, devising alternative approaches will be quite a challenge. As much as we would like to eliminate bias using objective measures, we realize that the process of comparing unique individuals is in some ways impossible. At a minimum, however, withholding the names of applicants from admissions committee members might begin to reduce the possibility of favoritism. Additionally, administrators should recruit and maintain a diverse community of people to serve on admission committees.

Beyond this, we know that past behavior is the best predictor of future behavior. Perhaps admissions committees should weigh an applicant's real-world experience as heavily as his or her academic performance. Favorable ratings could be given to those who have personally experienced poverty, discrimination, or homelessness; those who have demonstrated public service experience in demographically diverse communities; or those who have been or are willing to commit to working in underserved areas. Such behaviors and experiences are likely to reflect cultural sensitivity, increased interpersonal skills, and dedication to serving the individuals and communities with the greatest needs.

Applicants who are not accepted could receive individual feedback and guidance on how to improve their chances the following year. A school could even commit to individual students, giving them special consideration for the following year if certain tasks are completed. For students who are admitted but have not had access to the best educational environments, schools could offer summer programs and other bridging educational opportunities to provide remedial help.

For applicants who are accepted, medical schools must make a firm commitment to ensuring the success of their students. The following list of reforms would, we believe, help to address the needs of medical students.

— Make tutoring services available from the first day of medical school. Students should have easy and direct access to such aid. Faculty and administrators should pay attention to identifying students who are in need of academic support but might not yet know it.

— Establish and promote a mentoring system that includes upper-level classmates as well as pre-clinical, clinical, and community doctors who can guide students throughout medical school and into their careers.

— Offer psychological, group, and family support services throughout medical school.

— Appoint a staff member to advocate for and set up accommodations on behalf of students with disabilities or special needs.

— Recruit a diverse and sensitive group of staff and faculty at all levels of administration, including deans and student support services.

— Establish a teaching track as well as a research track for faculty promotions so that students are taught by people who have a vested interest in teaching them rather than in research.

— Utilize a more macroscopic focus in teaching about disease. Given the current level of specialization, a student in a cardiology class who asks a question about the impact of a heart malformation on lung function may not receive an adequate answer. A problem-based style of teaching, which requires a student to actively access a broader knowledge base, may be more effective than a didactic style.

— Allow students more choice in selecting the teachers they can best learn from.

— De-emphasize large lectures, and move to individual or small-group teaching, hands-on training, and different teaching modalities.

— Set up a clear list of expectations and goals for students. Knowledge bases and tasks should be prioritized and organized in clinically meaningful units, rather than being presented as an undifferentiated and unmanageable mass.

— Institute a strict pass/no pass system, which would help to eliminate competition among medical students. Optimal patient care requires all specialties of medicine to learn to work cooperatively, not competitively.

— Use exams not only as a way of evaluating students but also as a way of identifying gaps in knowledge. Give students the opportunity to demonstrate proficiency in a previously weak area.

— Move away from standardized, multiple-choice tests and toward tests that simulate reality, such as clinical case studies. This may help eliminate test questions focused on minutiae that are intended to shape the bell curve for grading purposes.

— Create a curriculum that is responsive to the changing needs and interests of students by supporting student-taught electives and including student representation on curricular design committees.

— Allow students some flexibility in their schedules to pursue research interests, engage in community projects, and attend to their personal lives.

— Provide funding for students to participate in multidisciplinary areas of research, to work in community projects, and to travel to student conferences, which can expand knowledge and forge networks among students who may feel isolated within their own schools.

— During the clinical years, work hours should be limited, and call schedules should be reasonable.

— Allow dedicated hours for teaching and studying.

— Clinical years should also be based on a pass/no pass system. Or, at a minimum, students should have clear, tangible, and attainable goals to fulfill in order to receive honors. Eliminate grading curves, and make it possible to achieve honors by other means, such as outstanding performance in clinics.

— Establish open office hours during which clinical professors are available to answer students' questions and help improve their clinical skills.

— Provide meal tickets when students must work long hours, don't have time to prepare meals, and cannot leave the hospital.

— Devise a system that doesn't put medical students into severe debt. Owing one or two hundred thousand dollars at the end of medical school is a huge burden and may influence a student's choice of specialization.

— Provide early and continuing professional career guidance so that students are exposed not only to a variety of medical specialties but also to other ways they can use their newfound skills and abilities to improve the world.

In summary, what we advocate is a humane system that will foster the training of humane physicians from all backgrounds. Society today requires doctors who are more diverse, approachable, and culturally sensitive, more creative and team-oriented, and less autocratic. Training such physicians requires an educational system that reflects these values.

Our reforms may appear naïve or impractical, but we believe that idealism is the necessary first step in the process of real change. If we, as a society, want the best physicians, we must make a commitment to the best training for them. Medical students of today need more than just the facts of medicine—like everyone else, they need well-rounded lives to allow them to flourish and become the types of doctors we would all want as our own: kind, compassionate, caring, knowledgeable, courageous, and, above all, human.

FURTHER READING

SOCIAL AND CULTURAL PERSPECTIVES ON MEDICINE

Becker, H. S. *Boys in White: Student Culture in Medical School.* Chicago: University of Chicago Press, 1961.

Fox, R. C. *Essays in Medical Sociology: Journeys into the Field.* New York: Wiley, 1979.

Wear, D. *Privilege in the Medical Academy: A Feminist Examines Gender, Race, and Power.* New York: Teachers College Press, 1997.

HISTORY OF MEDICINE

Gamble, V. N. *Making a Place for Ourselves: The Black Hospital Movement, 1920–1945.* New York: Oxford University Press, 1995.

Ludmerer, K. M. *Learning to Heal: The Development of American Medical Education.* New York: Basic Books, 1985.

———. *Time to Heal: American Medical Education from the Turn of the Century to the Era of Managed Care.* New York: Oxford University Press, 1999.

Starr, P. *The Social Transformation of American Medicine.* New York: Basic Books, 1982.

Walsh, M. R. *"Doctors Wanted, No Women Need Apply": Sexual Barriers in the Medical Profession, 1835–1975.* New Haven: Yale University Press, 1977.

Watson, W. H. *Against the Odds: Blacks in the Profession of Medicine in the United States.* New Brunswick, N.J.: Transaction Publishers, 1999.

PHYSICIAN NARRATIVES

Alvord, L. A., and E. C. Van Pelt. *The Scalpel and the Silver Bear.* New York: Bantam Books, 1999.

Conley, F. K. *Walking Out on the Boys.* New York: Farrar, Straus and Giroux, 1998.

DasGupta, S. *Her Own Medicine: A Woman's Journey from Student to Doctor.* New York: Ballantine, 1999.

Elders, J., and D. Chanoff. *Joycelyn Elders, M.D.: From Sharecropper's Daughter to Surgeon General of the United States of America.* New York: William Morrow, 1996.

Gawande, A. *Complications: A Surgeon's Notes on an Imperfect Science.* New York: Metropolitan Books, 2002.

Klass, P. *A Not Entirely Benign Procedure: Four Years as a Medical Student.* New York: G. P. Putnam, 1987.

Konner, M. *Becoming a Doctor: A Journey of Initiation in Medical School.* New York: Viking, 1987.

Marion, R. *Learning to Play God: The Coming of Age of a Young Doctor.* Reading, Mass.: Addison Wesley, 1991.

Remen, R. N. *Kitchen Table Wisdom: Stories That Heal.* New York: Riverhead Books, 1996.

Rothman, E. L. *White Coat: Becoming a Doctor at Harvard Medical School.* New York: William Morrow, 1999.

Verghese, A. *My Own Country: A Doctor's Story.* New York: Vintage Books, 1995.

MEDICAL STUDENTS: DEMOGRAPHICS, TRAINING, AND EXPERIENCES

Basco, W. T., Jr., S. B. Buchbinder, A. K. Duggan, and M. H. Wilson. "Relationship Between Primary Care Practices in Medical School Admission and the Matriculation of Underrepresented-Minority and Female Applicants." *Academic Medicine* 74, no. 8 (August 1999): 920–924.

DeVille, K. "Defending Diversity: Affirmative Action and Medical Education."

American Journal of Public Health 89, no. 8 (August 1999): 1256–1261.

Essex-Sorlie, D. "The Americans with Disabilities Act: II. Implications and Suggestions for Compliance for Medical Schools." *Academic Medicine* 69, no. 7 (July 1994): 525–534.

George, S. A. "Admission of Asian Americans to U.S. Medical Schools." *Academic Medicine* 73, no. 3 (March 1998): 226–227.

Lubitz, R. M., and D. D. Nguyen. "Medical Student Abuse During Third-Year Clerkships." *Journal of the American Medical Association* 275, no. 5 (1996): 414–416.

Robb, N. "Fear of Ostracism Still Silences Some Gay MDs, Students." *Canadian Medical Association Journal* 155, no. 7 (1996): 972–977.

CONTRIBUTORS

NUSHEEN AMEENUDDIN left Bangalore, India, for the American Midwest when she was a toddler. After completing her M.P.H. and M.D. at the University of Kansas, Nusheen began a pediatrics residency at the Mayo Clinic. She eventually hopes to combine a clinical practice with child advocacy work. Her most meaningful accomplishment has been performing the Hajj (pilgrimage to Mecca) with her parents while a senior medical student.

MARCIA VERENICE CASAS *"Recuerda, papagino, . . . cada momento que pasa es una nueva oportunidad para cambiar las cosas"* (Remember, *papagino*, . . . every day is a new chance to turn things around). Born a Mexicana, raised an American, Marcia found her way home in the years that followed. Passionate about international health, she hopes to specialize in emergency medicine and travel the world. Her greatest desires are to someday be a good wife, mother, and doctor.

SIMONE C. EASTMAN-UWAN was born in British Guyana to a single mother of two children. When she was fourteen, she immigrated to New York City to live with her grandmother. On graduating from Clara Barton High School in Brooklyn, she received a scholarship to Barnard College, where she majored in biological sciences. During her sophomore year, Simone became severely ill and was later diagnosed with sickle-cell anemia. She went on to attend Stanford University School of Medicine, where she was involved in sickle-cell anemia research and spoke to the medical community about living with a chronic, painful illness. After graduating in June 2001, Simone began a family practice residency.

KAY M. ERDWINN finished medical school in June 2000 and is currently devoting three to four years to other projects before beginning her residency. She is studying herbal medicine, psychoanalysis, shamanism, and energy medicine. She works as a crisis line volunteer and counselor at the El Dorado Women's Center and teaches a yoga class for large people.

UGO A. EZENKWELE, who was born in New York City, moved to rural Nigeria when he was nine years old. While there, he learned Igbo, a traditional Nigerian language. On returning to the United States, he attended high school at the United Nations International School in Manhattan. Ugo attended college and medical school at Johns Hopkins University, where he also obtained a master's degree in public health. Later he earned a Fulbright scholarship to help establish an injury surveillance system in the Caribbean. Ugo recently finished his emergency medicine residency at the University of Pennsylvania and is now an assistant professor of emergency medicine at New York University/Bellevue Hospital Center.

TISTA GHOSH, originally from Indiana, attended Indiana University Medical School. She is now a resident in a combined program in internal and preventive medicine and plans a career in international health.

HEATHER GOFF grew up in Essex, Connecticut, and then moved to Pennsylvania to attend Swarthmore College. She graduated from New York Medical College in 2002 and is now in a psychiatry residency program at Yale. She plans to specialize in child and adolescent psychiatry and would like to combine that with a life of teaching, writing, and family.

KAREN E. HERZIG, never a medical student, obtained her Ph.D. in health psychology at the University of California San Francisco, where she is currently a researcher. At the invitation of Kevin Takakuwa, Karen joined in preparation of the book; she coedited the stories, coauthored the non-story parts, and, ironically, conceived the book's title.

LAINIE HOLMAN was born in Stillwater, Oklahoma, during the Summer of Love. She did her undergraduate work at Antioch College in Yellow Springs, Ohio. After graduating from the Medical College of Ohio, she began a combined residency in pediatrics and physical medicine and rehabilitation at Cincinnati Children's Medical Center.

KAREN C. KIM was born at Stanford Hospital, raised in Los Angeles and the San Francisco Bay Area, attended college on the East Coast, and now spends a good number of days each week in a building attached to Stanford Hospital. In college, she majored in women's studies, with emphases in social anthropology and African history. In medical school, Karen has been involved with a project on physician activism and established a lecture series based on the work of Physicians for Social Responsibility and the role of physicians in furthering human rights and justice.

PAUL M. LANTOS, raised in Portland, Connecticut, graduated from the University of Connecticut School of Medicine, where he is currently a resident in a combined internal medicine and pediatrics program. Paul has secured a fellowship in infectious diseases at Harvard Medical School. He aspires to a career that will combine tropical medicine and international health.

RACHEL UMI LEE was born in Seoul, Korea, and raised in San Diego, California. She graduated from New York Medical College and is now an internal medicine resident at the Naval Medical Center in San Diego. Rachel's experiences include volunteering at a local homeless shelter and on a medical mission to the Yucatán in Mexico, which have cultivated a passion to work with underserved communities in the United States or abroad.

DAVID MARCUS is a board-certified psychiatrist with both clinical and research interests in Tourette syndrome, ADHD, and obsessive-compulsive disorder. In 2001, he completed a National Institutes of Health–sponsored postdoctoral fellowship, which taught him how to design and implement clinical drug trials. David now practices psychiatry in the Los Angeles area.

ROBERT "LAME BULL" MCDONALD was raised in Los Angeles and attended medical school at the University of Washington. He has been involved in the Medicine Wheel Society, an organization for Native American medical students and those interested in Native health issues. The organization's activities included performing sports physicals for Native American high school students, checking blood pressures at local powwows, hosting a yearly elders' dinner, and managing a street clinic for homeless American Indian people. "Hoka Hey!" the title of McDonald's story, is a Lakota term that translates literally as "Hold fast. There is more!"

TRESA MUIR MCNEAL grew up in Sanger, Texas, and now lives in Temple, Texas. She graduated from the Texas A&M University System Health Science Center College of Medicine. She is a resident in internal medicine and pediatrics at Scott and White Memorial Hospital, affiliated with Texas A&M. Tresa and her husband have recently been introduced to parenthood and its pleasures.

EDDY V. NGUYEN was born in Saigon, Vietnam. He immigrated to the United States in 1980 and settled in Santa Ana, California. He attended the University of California at Los Angeles and majored in biochemistry as an undergraduate. He graduated from medical school at Stanford University and is a resident in ophthalmology at the Jules Stein Eye Institute at UCLA Medical Center.

THAO NGUYEN, the oldest of three children, left Vietnam as a ten-year-old to come to the United States. She attended college at Oberlin in Ohio and attained honors in neuroscience. After finishing medical school at the University of California at Davis, she completed a residency program in family practice in Santa Rosa, California.

"LINDA PALAFOX," who chose to remain anonymous because of possible repercussions faced by alcoholics in the medical profession, continues her medical training as a family practice resident.

AKILESH PALANISAMY was born in Tamil Nadu, India, and came to the United States in 1988. He graduated from the University of California at San Francisco School of Medicine and began residency training in family practice at the San Jose Medical Center. Akilesh's interests are in end-of-life care, alternative medicine, and applied kinesiology.

ANITA RAMSETTY moved from St. Vincent and the Grenadines to attend college in Florida. She graduated from medical school in 2000 and from an internal medicine residency in 2003 at the University of Florida. Anita is now a fellow in endocrinology at Stanford University.

NICK RUBASHKIN was born and raised in a small town in Maine. He is currently a clinical student at Stanford University, where he recently completed a master's degree in social and cultural anthropology. He envisions a career on the border between social activism and medicine.

KEVIN M. TAKAKUWA graduated from medical school and is now a senior resident in emergency medicine at the Hospital of the University of Pennsylvania. He is currently writing another book.

MELANIE M. WATKINS graduated from Stanford University School of Medicine in 2003. She is currently a resident in obstetrics/gynecology at the University of California San Francisco and plans to work with the underserved. Melanie enjoys motivational speaking and would like to be a physician and writer. She has been profiled in *USA Today, Chicken Soup for the Single's Soul,* and *This Side of Doctoring: Reflections from Women in Medicine.*

ACKNOWLEDGMENTS

Kevin would like to thank the following individuals:

Drs. Kay M. Erdwinn, Jonathan M. Metzl, Stephen R. Smith, and Linda Ware for providing early, invaluable editorial assistance.

Drs. Kathryn Radke, Thomas Jue, Larry Hjelmeland, Shelley Chavoor, Amy Ernst, Steven Weiss, Jeanine Cogan, Margaret Carr, Christina Trevino, and Martha Hoopes for demonstrating kindness and humanity.

All of the American Medical Student Association representatives who forwarded to their classmates my e-mails requesting submissions for this book.

Genevieve F. Coutroubis and John F. Karpinski for their continuous support of this project.

At the University of California Press, Naomi Schneider for her enthusiastic and patient advocacy of this project, and Dore Brown and Mary Renaud for their careful work on the manuscript and production of this book.

.　.　.　.　.

In addition, Nick would like to thank the following people for their inspiration and support of this project:

At Stanford, I am grateful to the Arts and Humanities Medical Scholars program for funding historical research for the book; to Dr. R. Ruth Linden for advice, guidance, and conversation; to Dr. Ron Garcia, the Center of Excellence, and all the FACES speakers; to Tommy Lee Woon for inspiring the FACES program and for his endless ability to listen; to Ann Banchoff, Tim

Stanton, and my PRISMS cohort; and to Dr. Elliot Wolfe for continued encouragement to follow an individual path.

Thanks to my undergraduate adviser and friend, Amy Agigian (and Bob and Max!)—few others have been so influential in my personal and political development; and to Jyl Lynn Felman for the gift of free expression through the written word.

Thanks also to my dear friends Iram Qidwai and Jeannie Chang, co-founders of the FACES program in the medical school and partners in political change; to Nghe Yang for being my friend across the street; to Susanne Martin-Herz, my co-counseling partner and friend, for giving me the time to process; to Abigail Myers for always making me laugh; to Allison Wolf for changing and growing together; to my boys: Stephan Paschalides for his emotional beacon, Stephen Yosifon for his free-spirited nature, John Houghtling for attitude, and Richard Solomon for watching my stars. Thanks as well to the crew at IHPS—Richard Bae, Joanna Dearlove, Josh Dunsby, Gabriela Soto Laveaga, Meredith Nixon, Meighan Schreiber, Ryo Shohara—for all the supportive lunch sessions.

To my parents, Michael and Susan Rubashkin, activists in their own right—without your love and support, I would not be where I am. Thanks to the rest of my family for their love, especially my godmother, Mary Ann Collins.

To my dear boyfriend and fellow author, Drew Banks—you have been everything during this project: mentor, advocate, therapist, editor, and lover. Full moons forever.

Thanks to my late grandmother, Veronica Josephine Courtemanche, who once told me a story about being exposed to toxic fumes while working at a factory. She reported the incident, but the management refused to believe her story. In conclusion, she pointed her finger at me and said, "Don't forget that gay people aren't the only people in the world who are discriminated against." My work on this book is dedicated to her memory.

. . . . .

Finally, Karen would like to make the following acknowledgments:

Thank you to Barbara Gerbert, my colleague at the University of California San Francisco, for reviewing an early draft and providing ongoing enthusiasm and encouragement. Thanks also to David Lee for helpful advice throughout the process. Last but not least, thanks to Kevin Takakuwa for dragging me, kicking and screaming, into this project, for teaching me more about medical school than I ever hoped to know, and for paying the phone bills for all our hours-long, bicoastal editing, writing, and revising sessions over the past three years. Without Kevin's vision, commitment to the work, and sheer tenacity, this book would have remained merely another great idea.

PHOTO CREDITS

Nusheen Ameenuddin / © Syed Ameenuddin
Marcia Verenice Casas / © Rachel Mory
Simone C. Eastman-Uwan / © Aniekan Uwan
Kay M. Erdwinn / © Pro-Image Photography
Ugo A. Ezenkwele / © Dara Scott
Tista Ghosh / © Randy J. Shefman
Heather Goff / © Jennifer Philpott
Lainie Holman / © Mary Kay Smith
Karen C. Kim / © Christopher Hernandez
Paul M. Lantos / © Daniel Lantos
Rachel Umi Lee / © Helen Lin
David Marcus / © Mohsin Shah
Robert "Lame Bull" McDonald / © Kathy McDonald
Tresa Muir McNeal / © Richard Muir
Eddy V. Nguyen / © Mike Ghaly
Akilesh Palanisamy / © Ashok Swamy
Anita Ramsetty / © Mark A. Eckert
Nick Rubashkin / © Karren Baker
Kevin M. Takakuwa / © Genevieve Coutroubis
Melanie M. Watkins / © Ian Suydam

COMPOSITOR: Impressions Book and Journal Services, Inc.
TEXT: 10/15 Janson
DISPLAY: Orator
PRINTER AND BINDER: Sheridan Books, Inc.